OXFORD MEDICAL PUBLICATIONS

Prescribing in primary care

Prescribing in primary care

Oxford General Practice Series • 42

Edited by

F. D. Richard Hobbs

Professor and Head of General Practice,
University of Birmingham, Birmingham, UK

and

Colin P. Bradley

Professor of General Practice,
University College Cork, Cork, Ireland

Oxford : New York : Tokyo
OXFORD UNIVERSITY PRESS
1998

Oxford University Press, Great Clarendon Street, Oxford OX2 6DP
Oxford New York
Athens Auckland Bangkok Bogota Bombay Buenos Aires
Calcutta Cape Town Dar es Salaam Delhi Florence Hong Kong
Istanbul Karachi Kuala Lumpur Madras Madrid Melbourne
Mexico City Nairobi Paris Singapore Taipei Tokyo Toronto Warsaw
and associated companies in
Berlin Ibadan

Oxford is a trade mark of Oxford University Press

Published in the United States
by Oxford University Press Inc., New York

© Richard Hobbs, Colin Bradley & the contributors listed on p. xiii, 1988

A catalogue record for this book is available from the British Library

Library of Congress Cataloging in Publication Data
Prescribing in primary care / edited by F. D. Richard Hobbs and Colin P. Bradley.
(Oxford general practice series 42) (Oxford medical publications)
Includes bibliographical references.
1. Drugs—Prescribing. 2. Primary care (Medicine)
3. Drugs—Prescribing—Great Britain. 4. Primary care (Medicine)
—Great Britain. 5. National Health Service (Great Britain)
I. Hobbs, Richard, F. D. II. Bradley, Colin P. III. Series.
IV. Series: Oxford medical publications.
[DNLM: 1. Prescriptions, Drug. 2. Primary Health Care—Great Britain.
3. Drug Industry—Great Britain. W1 OX55 no. 42 1998 / QV 748 P9325 1998]
RM138.P726 1998 362.1'782—dc21 97–39639

ISBN 0 19 262687 6

Typeset by Jayvee, Trivandrum, India
Printed in Great Britain by
Biddles Ltd, Guildford & King's Lynn

CONTENTS

FOREWORD

Professor Sir Michael Drury

The achievements of the pharmaceutical industry would be sure to figure in any list of the scientific innovations of the twentieth century. Their effect upon disease rendering some preventable, some curable, and others tolerable has been enormous. The advent of a bewildering range of drugs with their capacity to do good, and sometimes harm, has lead to a spate of publications, books, scientific articles, and monthly and weekly journals. These have concentrated mostly upon describing the actions and interactions of individual drugs, their dose range, and the ways in which they are packaged and presented. These are useful and important tools for the doctor, especially the general practitioner whose range of drugs with which he must be familiar is so much greater than that of the specialist physician. All of this has contributed to prescribing becoming one of the most powerful tools in the armamentarium of the general practitioner.

However, every doctor now recognizes there is much more to prescribing than the ordering of a drug to treat the patient's problem. The very act of prescribing, and often even more so of non-prescribing, has considerable and measurable therapeutic significance. The pattern of a doctor's prescribing will influence the behaviour of patients and their families. The cost of a doctor's prescribing will affect expenditure upon other services within the practice and cumulatively on a national scale. The choice between alternative therapies and orthodox medicines has become an important factor in judgements about cost, safety, and efficacy.

None of these topics has gone unnoticed by the researcher and the commentator, but for the thinking doctor who wants to know more about such matters gaining access to them has not been easy. That is one reason why I welcome this book and recommend it so strongly. It covers the widest range of topics, each one of which is carefully referenced for source and further reading.

That is not to imply that this is a book only for the researcher. No one who prescribes, and can therefore have a profound influence upon the progress of illness, the behaviour of illness, and the well being of the Health Service should disregard the messages contained. Professors Hobbs and Bradley, together with their team of contributors, have produced a book which should make a considerable contribution to the quality of primary care. I hope it will be widely read.

PREFACE

Richard Hobbs

Prescribing treatment is a significant, perhaps the most significant, function of primary care physicians in all healthcare systems. At its most pure definition, it describes the giving of authoritative advice or instruction. As such, prescribing covers the management options considered by a physician to be most appropriate for individual patients. It therefore remains the case that physicians today will 'prescribe' a course of physical therapy or lifestyle modification. However, although it may be accurate to describe the offering of such management options as prescribing, the term has come to be synonymous with the prescription of medication.

This is not altogether unexpected, since the majority of consultations in developed healthcare systems will result in a prescription for a drug. Furthermore, the activity of prescribing medication consumes a significant proportion of healthcare expenditure in most countries. In the UK, slightly over 10% of total healthcare expenditure has been drug costs since the inception of the NHS in 1948 (Chew, 1995). In a sense, it is remarkable that this proportion of total expenditure has remained relatively constant over nearly 50 years in view of the huge growth in biologically active treatments since 1948, with many of the recent very expensive drugs being developed only during the latter years.

It is the growth of effective and safe drug treatments that has transformed the practice of medicine during the past half century. Without active treatments for potentially fatal conditions, such as diabetes, or common chronic problems, such as hypertension, asthma, or arthritis, it would be difficult to contemplate modern medicine as a service that encompasses public health as well as personal healthcare. The special place drugs have established in modern medicine has, unsurprisingly, resulted in their dominating the management decisions of modern physicians. This book therefore deals with the modern interpretation of prescribing; the action of physicians in issuing therapeutic medications.

The sheer scale of prescribing within primary healthcare may be gauged by the 473 million prescriptions issued by UK general practitioners each year, at a 1995 cost of £3681 million; and the 40–72% of all GP consultations which result in a prescription being issued (Webb and Lloyd, 1994; Government Statistical Service, 1996). However, prescribing remains a highly complex activity: patient expectations about needing a prescription do not often correlate with actual prescribing by doctors (most studies show that doctors issue prescriptions on more occasions than patients expect); disparate pressures exist on GPs, from a variety of sources, to prescribe more and yet other influences exist to prescribe less; and proxy measures of prescribing quality may be high levels of prescribing in one condition, but underprescribing in another (such as benzodiazepine versus inhaled steroid prescribing). Such prescribing issues are germane to all healthcare systems and yet many of the processes and influences surrounding prescribing are ill understood.

Given the importance of the subject, it is surprising that there is so little published on prescribing as an activity. A wealth of literature exists on drugs themselves, in terms of their actions, indications, and adverse effects. Many original papers consider new indications for new or existing drugs. The randomized control trial in medicine has been particularly associated with the development of novel therapeutic compounds. However, in contrast, the actions of physicians in offering treatment, the actions of prescribing, have received much less attention in both original research and descriptive literature. Since prescribing is such an important function of physicians, particularly primary care physicians, and the act of prescribing remains such a significant cost to the healthcare system, this is all the more surprising.

This book aims to inform a wider audience on the subject of drug prescribing. The book covers a wide range of areas from how drugs are developed, through the licensing of drugs to the ways they are marketed to physicians. The chapter on how doctors choose drugs explores this significantly under-researched physician activity. Further chapters consider how doctors can approach more rational prescribing, with chapters on the implications of the NHS reforms and on how doctors need to adapt their prescribing behaviours to comply with the requirements of the reformed NHS. The importance of drug costs is considered in a chapter on how to evaluate therapeutic expenditure with the framework of economic analysis.

Since the physician is not the only source of medication, the book also includes sections on the pharmacist, as the dispenser of prescribed medication and the advisor on over-the-counter medicines. This book does not consider the use of individual drugs, as this material is amply covered elsewhere; however, a chapter on homoeopathy which mentions some specific remedies has been included. Such alternative medicine has become a more popular option considered by patients in the latter part of the twentieth century. The relative paucity of information available to the physician on homoeopathy warranted our including this chapter.

We hope the reader will gain new information and new insights into this important clinical activity. Much of the text relates to the legislative position of prescribing as it operates in the UK. However, the book has much of relevance to an international audience since many of the external influences on prescribing operate, to at least some extent, in most developed health systems. Furthermore, many of the chapters consider topics that are not country specific.

This book should be of value to most physicians operating in primary care, to doctors or undergraduates training for primary care, to allied professions involved in the primary prescribing process, particularly pharmacists, and to all those involved in seeking to regulate or influence prescribing.

References

Chew, R. (1995). *Compendium of health statistics.* Office of Health Economics, London.

Government Statistical Service (1996). *Statistics of prescriptions dispensed in the Family Health Services Authorities: England 1985 to 1995.*

Webb, S., Lloyd, M. (1994). Prescribing and referral in general practice: a study of patients' expectations and doctors actions. *British Journal of General Practice,* **44**, 165–9.

CONTRIBUTORS

Nicholas Bateman, Consultant Physician and Reader in Therapeutics, University of Newcastle upon Tyne

Christine Bond, Senior Lecturer, Department of General Practice and Primary Care, University of Aberdeen

Alison Blenkinsopp, Director of Education and Research, Department of Medicines Management, University of Keele

Colin Bradley, Professor of General Practice, University College Cork

Yvonne Carter, Professor of Primary Care and General Practice, St. Bartholomew's and the Royal London

Petra Denig, Senior Lecturer in Drug Utilization Research, University of Groningen, The Netherlands

Alan Earl-Slater, Senior Lecturer in Health Economics, Department of Medicines Management, University of Keele

John Ferguson, Medical Director, Prescription Pricing Authority

Sheila Greenfield, Lecturer in Medical Sociology, University of Birmingham

Richard Hobbs, Professor of General Practice, University of Birmingham

Mollie Hunton, General Practitioner and Homeopathic Physician, Stourbridge

Michael Langman, Dean and Professor of Medicine, University of Birmingham

Frank Leach, North Western Regional Drug Information Centre, Manchester

David Millson, Drug Team Leader, Zeneca Pharmaceuticals, Macclesfield, Cheshire

Ross Taylor, Senior Lecturer in General Practice, University of Aberdeen

Tom Walley, Professor of Clinical Pharmacology, University of Liverpool

Andy Wearn, Lecturer in General Practice, University of Birmingham

Frank Wells, Director, Department of Medicine, Science and Technology, Association of the British Pharmaceutical Industry

ABBREVIATIONS AND ACRONYMS

ABPI	Association for the British Pharmaceutical Industry
ACE	angiotensin converting enzyme
AE	adverse event
ASTRO PU	age, sex and temporary resident prescribing unit
BNF	*British National Formulary*
CANDA	computer assisted NDA
COMPASS	Computerized On-line Monthly Prescribing Analysis for Science and Stewardship
CPMP	Committee on Proprietary Medicinal Products
CRO	clinical research organization
CTC	clinical trials certificate
CTX	clinical trial exemption
DDD	defined daily dose
DHA	District Health Authority
DM	disease management
DMI	Drug Master Index (UK DoH)
DoH	Department of Health (UK)
DSS	decision support systems
eBNF	*Electronic British National Formulary*
EC	European Commission
ED1	efficacy decision point

EMEA	European Agency for the Evaluation of Medicinal Products
EU	European Union
FDA	Food and Drug Administration (USA)
FHS	Family Health Service
FHSA	Family Health Service Authority
FPC	Family Practitioner Committee
GCP	good clinical practice
GMP	good manufacturing practice
GPRD	General Practice Research Database (formerly VAMP)
GSL	general sales list
IMS	Intercontinental Medical Statistics
IND	Investigational New Drug
INR	International normalized ratio
IPA	indicative prescribing amount
IPS	indicative prescribing scheme
ISE	integrated summary of efficacy
ISS	integrated summary of safety
KPI	Karnofsky Performance Index
LMC	Local Medical Committee
MASC	Medical Advisers Support Centre
MCA	Medicines Control Agency (UK)
MPV	medical practice variation
NCE	new chemical entity
NDA	new drug application
NDTI	National Disease and Therapeutic Index
NHP	Nottingham Health Profile
NHS	National Health Service (UK)
NIC	net ingredient cost
NPF	Nurse Prescribers' Formulary
NRTs	nicotine replacement therapies
NSAIDs	non-steroidal anti-inflammatory drugs
OTC	over the counter
P	pharmacy medicine

PACT	*Prescribing Analysis and Cost*
PAI	pre-approval inspection
PARS	Prescribing Audit Reports
PDD	prescribed daily dose
POM	prescription only medicine
PPA	Prescription Pricing Authority (UK)
PPRS	Pharmaceutical Price Regulation Scheme
PRODIGY	*Prescribing RatiOnally with Decision Support In General Practice StudY*
PU	prescribing unit
QA	quality assurance
QALY	quality adjusted life year
QoL	quality of life
RCT	randomized controlled trial
RMO	Regional Medical Officers
SIP	sickness impact profile
SOP	standard operating procedure
SPA	Scottish Prescribing Analysis
SSRI	selective serotonin reuptake inhibitor
TPP	target product profile
WHO	World Health Organization

CHAPTER ONE

Attempts to influence prescribing in the UK

Colin Bradley and Richard Hobbs

The prescribing of drugs has always been central to the function of the general practitioner and indeed to the role of all healers in all societies. One of the key components of the Medical Act of 1858 was to limit the right to prescribe drugs to those who were properly trained and hence recognized as being entitled to describe themselves as doctors. Talcott Parson's (1952) sociological description of what makes a doctor highlighted the central role of prescribing in the activity of doctoring. In his model of the sick role, the patient's responsibilities included one of seeking medical attention. One of the key responsibilities of the doctor was to provide a vindication of the patient's right to be treated as ill, of which the most visible manifestation is the issuing of a prescription.

This concept of every illness requiring a treatment and treatment being virtually synonymous with the prescribing of a drug is very strong in our culture even today. Studies of the frequency of prescribing illustrate how powerful this notion is. All such studies have shown that more than half the patients consulting a doctor will leave with a prescription (Stimpson and Webb, 1975; Cartwright and Anderson, 1981; Webb and Lloyd, 1994). Some studies have recorded rates of over 90% of consultations resulting in a prescription (Wilkin et al., 1987). International comparison suggest that in some countries the situation may be even more marked with virtually 100% of all consultations resulting in a prescription, often for more than one medicament (DeMaesener, 1989).

In the days before the advent of modern scientifically based medicine, medical practice was much more heavily reliant on the placebo effect which is difficult, if not impossible, to achieve without appearing to prescribe a medicine (Spiro, 1986). It was argued that little harm came of this policy since medicines used were not 'very strong' and the benefits achieved disproportionately great. Clearly, such views were inaccurate as some of the treatments of the pre-scientific era were potentially harmful; however, such complacency is no longer tolerable when we understand so much more about both the harmful and the beneficial effects of today's potent medicines. The adverse effects of medication were probably most graphically illustrated to the professions, the pharmaceutical industry, the government and, indeed, the general public by the thalidomide tragedy. The world-wide response to this catastrophe has been a tightening up in the regulation of medicines.

One result of this regulation has been to require the prescriber to be much clearer about the justification for medicine use in any given case, with an expectation that he or she prescribe with a complete awareness of the risks involved. This expectation is reinforced by the threat of successful medico-legal action against a doctor who is deemed to have failed to have exercised due care in the use of medicines. This is not to say that the problem of medicines being used inappropriately primarily for their placebo effect is no longer with us, but such action is now much more subtle (Brody, 1977). What is distinctly different is the much greater role of regulatory authorities in prescribing, through their review of all new medicines and their licensing of only those found to be safe and effective, and then only for prescribed purposes (see also Chapter 3).

In addition to controls on the availability and indications for medicines, to ensure their safe and effective use, has come the realization that medicines' uses must also be as economical as possible, particularly in countries where the state meets much or all of the cost of prescription drugs consumed. In the UK various attempts have been made to achieve this. Viewed from a historical perspective, these efforts have involved persuasion, education, or trying to get physicians to be more economical in their prescribing, and more prescriptive or legislative approaches to the problem.

Educational limitations on GP prescribing in the UK

From the start of the NHS, the amount of money spent on drugs exceeded expectations, and actions to tackle this were initiated (Dunlop *et al.*, 1952). The earliest legislative attempt to control the drugs bill in the UK was the introduction of a prescription charge, the very threat of which so affronted Aneurin Bevan, the architect of the NHS, with its principle of a service to be free at the point of use, that he resigned (Webster, 1991). The prescription charge was in fact introduced not by the government of which he was part, but by the incoming Conservative administration.

Even in those early days more subtle approaches were also made, and within a few years of the establishment of the NHS, certain Ministry of Health medical staff, known as Regional Medical Officers (RMOs), were given the task of visiting those general practices noted in the prescribing statistics to be exceeding local prescribing expenditure norms. This was the approach preferred by Bevan, who sought agreement to the principle of being able to discipline doctors whose prescribing was considered extravagant. The expectation was that such visits would encourage doctors to review their prescribing practice and, hopefully, change to a pattern that was closer to the norm and, hence, less expensive. The limited evidence available suggests this approach was moderately successful (Tricker, 1977), but developments since suggest that the activity was not sufficient to meet the government's need to contain primary care prescribing costs. During the 1990s, the functions of the RMOs in providing advice and feedback on prescribing to general practitioners has become the responsibility of pharmaceutical or medical advisers at health authorities (see Chapter 7).

Other educational approaches have concentrated on the provision to prescribers of information about drugs from sources independent of the pharmaceutical industry, who have always been recognized as a major source of influence on doctors. Thus doctors in the UK receive, at the government's expense, three publications with drug information. These are the *British National Formulary* published by the British Medical Association and the Royal Pharmaceutical Association of Great Britain; the *Prescribers' Journal* published by Stationery Office; and the *Drug and Therapeutics Bulletin* published by the Consumers' Association. In addition, prescribers in England and Wales receive the *MeReC Bulletin* from the Medicines Resource Centre and Scottish prescribers receive an equivalent publication from the Scottish Medicines Resource Centre. Other regional and local prescribing advisers and drug information units also send prescribers additional information at their own discretion.

In addition to this background information, prescribers throughout the UK are also provided with feedback on the pattern of their own prescribing from agencies who handle, on the government's behalf, the payment of pharmacists for prescriptions dispensed. As recommended in 1977 by Tricker, this data on drugs dispensed and paid for has been linked electronically to prescribing doctors via their unique prescribing code number. This data is analysed and presented to prescribing doctors in the form of, usually quarterly, reports showing how the doctor compares to local and national averages and how prescribing in various therapeutic categories is changing over time.

In England this is provided by the Prescription Pricing Authority as PACT (Prescribing Analysis and CosT) data, which is described in more detail in Chapter 7. In Scotland this is provided by the Prescribing Division of the Home and Health Department as SPA (Scottish Prescribing Analysis) data, in Wales by the Welsh Office as PARS (Prescribing Audit Reports) and in Northern Ireland by the Drug Utilization Research Unit as a COMPASS (Computerized On-line Monthly Prescribing Analysis for Science and Stewardship) Report. Although they were originally described as part of an educational initiative, with the introduction of the concept of 'drug budgets' and the continuing 'downward pressure on prescribing costs', these various reports are also part of a more subtle and more proscriptive campaign to contain the drugs bill. Such perceptions are reinforced by the fact that the reports all concentrate heavily on cost information, and particularly on information where costs are high.

Legislative limitations on GP prescribing in the UK

Other more legislative approaches in the UK include the introduction in April 1985 of the 'limited list' which restricted prescribing on the NHS in seven therapeutic areas to relatively few generic drugs. The seven categories of drugs affected by this initiative were antacids, laxatives, cough and cold remedies, analgesics for mild to moderate pain, vitamins, tonics and benzodiazepines. Thirty-one preparations, all of them exclusively generic versions of the drugs within these groups, were deemed sufficient to meet all clinical needs; all others were blacklisted. Similar lists of drugs which are either prohibited (negative lists) or to which prescribing must be restricted (positive lists) within state healthcare systems exist in Belgium, Greece, France, Ireland, Italy, Luxembourg, Portugal, and Spain. (Bangeman and Flynn, 1993)

Although quite fiercely resented by UK general practitioners at the time of its imposition, this restriction has, in the longer term, been viewed by some as possibly even beneficial (Taylor and Bond, 1985). A major source of the practitioner resentment was the lack of any prior consultation with the profession as to what might or might not meet real clinical need. However, since the introduction of the blacklist an advisory group has been set up to advise the Minister on what might or might not be included in the list and the number of preparations allowable within these groups had risen from the original 31 to 129 by February 1986.

Despite an apparent undertaking that this was to be a one-off manoeuvre, a further proposal to limit prescribing in a further 10 therapeutic areas was made in November 1992. These groups were antidiarrhoeal drugs, drugs for allergic disorders, hypnotics and anxiolytics, appetite suppressants, drugs for vaginal and vulval conditions, contraceptives, drugs used in anaemia, topical antirheumatics, drugs acting on the ear and nose, and drugs acting on the skin. The impact of this limited list has been much more muted. So far in only 5 of these 10 categories have drugs been blacklisted, and in these 5 areas the total number blacklisted is still only 63.

The pharmaceutical industry in the UK have been resentful of this approach to restricting prescribing, because the government has made it clear that one of the principal criteria for deciding between drugs will be cost. For example, in the case of topical NSAIDS, preparations below a certain price per 100 g were not blacklisted and those above were. The industry consider this to be 'reference pricing' by the back door, i.e. the placement of a price ceiling on what the NHS will pay for a drug (Reekie, 1995). The system of reference pricing, in which insurers will pay a proportion of the cost of drugs only up to a certain 'reference price' and any shortfall in the actual price has to be made up by the patient, already exists in other countries, most notably Germany.

The Health Committee of the House of Commons set up to enquiry into the NHS drugs bill has supported a different approach and suggested instead the introduction of a 'white list' (Health Committee, 1994). In contrast to a blacklist which lists the drugs not to be used, the white list would name those drugs to be used in preference to the host of those available. This is similar to the idea of a 'national formulary' in the sense in which the word formulary is now used (see Chapter 8 for details). The Committee proposed that all drugs at launch (following the completion of the assessments of safety, efficacy and quality required

4

for licensing) would automatically be white listed, but that after 5 years they would be reviewed and those drugs found to be less effective, or more expensive with no therapeutic advantages, would then be excluded. They further suggested that the evidence for effectiveness might be systematically evaluated by the Cochrane Centre in Oxford which was set up to evaluate clinical trials. A key difference between this white list and the current blacklist would be the provision of a mechanism whereby a doctor would still be allowed, exceptionally, to prescribe a drug not on the list. This mechanism would involve seeking the prior permission of the health authority medical or pharmaceutical adviser.

One obvious way in which prescribing costs could be reduced is to make generic prescribing or dispensing obligatory or, at least, make generic dispensing the default position, requiring doctors to override this default if they have some reason why a generic preparation will not suffice. This option has been suggested many times by successive government reviews of prescribing in the NHS and the idea of generic substitution (i.e. the right of the pharmacist to automatically substitute a generic form of the drug prescribed unless the doctor indicates that this is not to occur) has been introduced in some healthcare systems. These options have always been rejected in the UK; however, it appears that the potential economies of generic prescribing may be being achieved by other means since generic prescribing rates in the UK have risen steadily over the past decade, presumably under the influence of these other pressures.

Generic prescribing was once again highlighted in the document introducing the Indicative Prescribing System in 1990. This scheme, described more fully in Chapter 8, is a good illustration of an eclectic approach to changing prescribing practice, containing elements of both legislative and educational approaches. As well as leading to the establishment of mechanisms for setting doctors prescribing budgets, the system also expanded the RMO-type role with the introduction of prescribing advisors at health authorities and added a further source of independent prescribing advice in the form of the *MeReC Bulletin* (see above).

An interesting new attempt to influence primary physicians came in the form of the General Practitioner Fundholding Scheme, which gave doctors more control over their own budgets but more responsibility for restricting the cost of their clinical activities, including prescribing, to remain within these budgets. A more limited version of the same approach has been available in the form of incentive schemes in which doctors do not take on the full responsibilities of fundholding activities, but can agree certain target savings in prescribing. If targets are achieved, this can lead to a partial rebate of the putative savings into the practice for other developments. Also within the Improving Prescribing document, which launched the Indicative Prescribing Scheme, was the threat of an expansion of the procedures for investigation of 'excessive' prescribing. Although at the time of the introduction of prescribing budgets—then called 'indicative prescribing amounts' because the word 'budget' was politically sensitive—there was a concern that the new mechanism for dealing with 'excessive prescribing' might be invoked for any doctor exceeding their budget. As has transpired, the mechanism for investigating 'excessive prescribing' has not been invoked very often and it is still largely a fail-safe mechanism which picks up on extreme cases, such as those where there are major problems with prescribing involving fraud being perpetrated by doctors or pharmacists.

Drugs play a central role in the delivery of modern primary care as they constitute the principal intervention for many problems presenting in primary care. Modern drugs require closer attention to the balance of safety and efficacy and also, because of their increasingly high relative cost, oblige the healthcare funders to make strenuous efforts to control prescribing expenditure to the minimum necessary to achieve optimum benefit at least cost. To achieve this balance through an independent profession, working within a contractual arrangement that is tightly specified and difficult to alter, presents a considerable challenge and has lead to a range of sophisticated and sometimes crude state-funded influences operating on the prescribing process and incorporating both educational and legislative elements.

References

Bangemann, M., Flynn, M. (1993). Communication to Council and Parliament on the outline of an industrial policy for the pharmaceutical sector in the European Community. *Bulletin of the European Union Community*, **93**, 718.

Brody, H. (1977). *Placebos and the philosophy of medicine.* University of Chicago Press, Chicago.

Cartwright, A., Anderson, R. (1981). *General practice revisited.* Tavistock, London.

DeMaesner, J. (1989). The functioning of 94 GP trainers: an exploratory study. PhD Thesis, State University, Ghent, Belgium.

Dunlop, D. M., Henderson, T. L., Inch, R. S. (1952). A survey of 17,301 prescriptions on Form EC10. *British Medical Journal*, **1**, 292–5.

House of Commons Health Committee (1994). *Second report into priority setting in the NHS: The NHS drugs budget.* HMSO, London.

Parsons, T. (1952). Social structure and dynamic process: The case of modern medical practice. In *The social system* by T. Parsons, Chapter 10. Tavistock, London.

Reekie, W. D. (1995). *Prescribing the price of pharmaceuticals.* Institute of Economic Affairs Health and Welfare Unit, London.

Spiro, H. M. (1986). *Doctors, patients and placebos.* Yale University Press, New Haven.

Stimpson, G., Webb, B. (1975). *Going to see the doctor. The consultation process in general practice.* Routledge and Kegan Paul, London.

Taylor, R. J., Bond, C. M. (1985). Limited list: limited effects? *British Medical Journal*, **291**, 518–20.

Tricker, R. I. (1977). Role of the DHSS in relation to the PPA. In *Report of the inquiry into the Prescription Pricing Authority*, Chapter 9, pp. 84–7. HMSO, London.

Webb, S., Lloyd, M. (1994). Prescribing and referral in general practice: a study of patients' expectations and doctors' actions. *British Journal of General Practice*, **44**, 165–9.

Webster, C. (1991). *Aneurin Bevan on the National Health Service*. Wellcome Unit for the History of Medicine, Oxford.

Wilkin, D., Hallam, L., Leavey, R., Metcalfe, D. (1987). Patterns of care. In *Anatomy of urban general practice*, Chapter 7. Tavistock, London.

CHAPTER TWO

National and international patterns of drug use

Ross Taylor

Drug utilization studies

Sources of data

Good data on drug utilization are not readily available. Data for commercial purposes are obtained by the pharmaceutical industry and associated bodies such as the Association of the British Pharmaceutical Industry (ABPI). These data may come from information on sales of medicines or from special studies by commercial survey organizations such as Intercontinental Medical Statistics (IMS). Apart from sales data, the other main source is operational data from general practice.

The UK has one of the most comprehensive databases in the world as a by-product of the need for the NHS to price every dispensed prescription for payment to pharmacists through the Prescription Pricing Authority (PPA) and its equivalent in Scotland (see Chapter 8). Although comprehensive in its coverage of the whole country, and informative in its ability to identify time trends and inter-regional variations, the huge PPA database is nonetheless far from perfect, because it was not designed for drug utilization studies. Its main deficiencies are that it contains only prescription data, with no indication of diagnosis or 'reason for prescription'; that it cannot distinguish acute from repeat prescriptions; and that individual prescriptions cannot be reliably assigned to individual doctors making inter-doctor comparison difficult. The system also cannot give the number of persons receiving a medicine as opposed to the number of prescriptions.

General practice microcomputer systems are capable of producing the kind of data which is missing from the PPA system, and are increasingly available, but are still far away from the level of accuracy and comprehensive national coverage which are available from PPA statistics. In most GP microcomputer systems it is possible to link prescribing with morbidity, giving some indication of the reason for a prescription, and to link prescriptions with persons whilst still preserving anonymity. This is important in studying the utilization of the many drugs, such as beta blockers, which can be used for a number of different indications (e.g. angina, anxiety, hypertension).

In the UK the General Practice Research (formerly VAMP) Database (GPRD), currently administered through the Department of Health (DoH) is the best known (Jick *et al.*, 1991, 1992), but there are others, including the continuous morbidity recording project operated by the Birmingham Research Unit of the Royal College of General Practitioners (Fleming and Fullarton, 1993) and parallel projects in Scotland (Taylor *et al.*, 1990; Whitelaw *et al.*, 1996) and Northern Ireland (Boydell *et al.*, 1995). As general practice microcomputer systems begin to cover the majority of the national population and as completeness and accuracy of data increases they are likely to become a major source of drug utilization data.

Nevertheless, it is important to realize the comparative limitations of drug utilization data. The main deficiency is that it is usually impossible to judge 'appropriateness'. For example, the consumption of H_2 antagonists might be similar per head of population in two different practices. It is theoretically possible that all the prescriptions issued by doctors in one practice are 'appropriate'—i.e. all for recognized indications such as peptic ulcer—and all the prescriptions issued by doctors in the second practice are 'inappropriate', with none of those who should receive H_2 antagonists actually receiving them.

The development of generally agreed international standards for 'appropriateness', and the development of databases which link prescribing data with explanatory data (e.g. morbidity) are therefore a major priority for drug utilization research (Tomson, 1991; Anis *et al.*, 1996). Even diagnosis-linked data will go only part of the way in explaining variation in drug utilization because 'diagnoses' vary in definition, accuracy and validity and, as is discussed later, morbidity may only be one factor (although a major one) in prescribing.

Apart from those already mentioned, there are diagnosis-linked drug utilization databases in the USA and Sweden (Strom, 1989) and there are a number of other sources of prescription-only data comparable to UK PPA data available in other countries (e.g. Norway, Spain, Sweden, USA), although these may not provide the same comprehensive national coverage as PPA. In the USA, in particular, more detailed and useful information is increasingly available from health systems such as Medicaid, and from large health maintenance organizations such as Kaiser Permanente. IMS is also a major provider of information to industry and government in both the USA and the UK. Its data come from a variety of sources including special sample surveys of GP prescribing, such as the National Disease and Therapeutic Index (NDTI) by IMS America Ltd, and similar quarterly surveys based on carbon copy prescription forms collected by co-operative samples of general practitioners in the UK and Ireland.

Units of measurement

In the UK, prescribing statistics have conventionally been presented in terms of three main parameters:

- number of items per patient
- cost per item
- cost per patient.

Cost generally indicates net ingredient cost (NIC). This does not include additional fees payable to pharmacists, which add about a further one-third to the total cost of the national drug bill. All of these measures are invalidated by the absence of any measure of quantity of drug prescribed. Number of items per patient is, perhaps, the least valid measurement. This is because if one doctor habitually issues prescriptions for one month's supply of an antihypertensive, say, while another favours a two month supply, the second doctor's item per patient rate will be half that of the first doctor's, even if they were supplying exactly the same quantities of medicine.

Cost per item suffers from the same problem, because it consists of two dimensions: the unit cost (expensiveness) of the medicine and the quantity of medicine supplied. Cost per patient is perhaps the best of these imperfect measurements for comparison between general practices, regions and nations, whereas the other measures may have some value for intra-practice analyses (see Chapter 8). Cost per patient might be less valid for short periods of time because of the quantity per item problem already outlined, but annual rates are likely to be more valid. Of course, drug consumption varies a great deal with age and with sex, so that age–sex specific rates would be best, but PPA data do not include age and sex of the patient.

The most meaningful unit of measurement currently available is the defined daily dose (DDD), originally developed in Scandinavia and now promoted under the auspices of the World Health Organization (WHO) (Lee and Bergman, 1989). The DDD is a standardized unit of volume for use in drug utilization studies. It is a notional unit which does not necessarily reflect the dose in which the drug in question might be used. It is usually the assumed average maintenance dose for the main indication of the drug (see Table 2.1).

Because the DDD does not always reflect actual clinical practice, another unit—the prescribed daily dose (PDD)—is sometimes used. This is based on the average daily dose actually prescribed in a representative sample of prescriptions. The PDD may be better for comparisons within countries, because it reflects the actual prescribing practice in that country. Dosage regimes vary considerably between countries, however, so that higher PDDs for drugs such as hydrochlorothiazide, diazepam, and oxazepam have been noted in the USA relative to Sweden (Lee and Bergman, 1989). The notional DDD therefore still seems best for international comparisons. Despite the deficiencies of the system (there are, for example, no DDDs for dermatological preparations) drugs of a similar class (e.g. NSAIDs) can be added together because DDDs are designed to be equipotent.

In comparisons of drug utilization by therapeutic grouping it is also difficult to ensure exact comparability. Different systems of classification are used (for example, within the UK itself there was a change in classification from the

Table 2.1 *Example of DDDs*

Drug	DDD
Amoxycillin	1 g
Atenolol	75 mg
Bendrofluazide	2.5 mg
Cimetidine	800 mg
Diclofenac	100 mg
Digoxin	0.25 mg
Frusemide	40 mg
Glyceryl trinitrate	5 mg
Ibuprofen	1.2 g
Nifedipine	30 mg
Paracetamol	3 g
Phenoxymethyl penicillin	2 g
Prednisolone	10 mg
Propranolol	160 mg
Ranitidine	300 mg
Temazepam	20 mg
Terfenadine	120 mg

Department of Health Drug Master Index (DMI) system to the *British National Formulary* (BNF) classification which can cause difficulties in comparing time trends).

It is not usually possible to distinguish acute from long-term use of a drug. Thus one could not say from PPA data how much erythromycin is being used long term for acne as opposed to its use in acute infections. Finally, most large drug databases are of prescribed medicines only. This creates difficulties for international comparison because there are widespread differences in the proportion of all medicines consumed in a country that are prescribed, as opposed to being directly purchased without prescription. Until recently, the UK was much more restrictive than many other countries. Now (see Chapter 10) increasing deregulation means that many potent drugs are available in the UK through either route. This creates increasing difficulties for comparative studies within the UK (because only prescription data can enter the PPA database) as well as between nations and increases dependence on overall sales data.

Looking for patterns in drug utilization

Time trends

There has been a steady upward trend in NHS spending on medicines over the years, but this has largely paralleled the general rise in gross NHS expenditure so that medicines expenditure has tended to absorb a fairly constant proportion (about 10%) of the total NHS budget.

A detailed analysis of prescribing was undertaken by the DoH for the Health Committee of the House of Commons (1994). This concluded that the trend in overall volume of prescription items had been upwards since the early 1960s, with the rate of increase rising since the mid-1980s, and the increases in the most recent years (4.8% in 1991 and 4.7% in 1992) being higher than at any time in the previous 10 years. This was the product of two effects:

- change in the size and age-mix of the population
- change in the average number of prescriptions per head of population.

Quoting directly from the DoH evidence,

Just under a seventh of the increase in volume between 1982 and 1992 can be explained by 'pure demography', i.e. an increase in the size of the population and, in particular, of the numbers of elderly people—elderly people receive more prescriptions per head than the rest of the population (19.3 in 1992 compared with 4.5 for children and 6.1 for adults under pension age).

The other six sevenths of the increase are explained by an increase in the average number of prescriptions per head. The average number of prescriptions per head for the population as a whole in 1992 was 8.2, compared with 5.0 in 1959 and 6.7 in 1982. Between 1982 and 1992 the percentage increase in the number of prescriptions per head for people of pension age was much higher than for the rest of the population: 44.5% compared with 13.3% for children and 8.0% for adults under pension age.

The reasons put forward by DoH for the increase in volume of prescribing are given in Box 2.1. Between 1982 and 1992 (at 1992 prices) the average net ingredient cost (NIC) per prescription also rose (see Table 2.2). Over the same period

---

Box 2.1 *Probable explanations for the increase in numbers of prescriptions per head 1982–1992 (DoH)*

- New types of drug therapy for conditions which were previously not treatable or could be treated only in hospital
- Marketing effort by manufacturers to increase awareness of new types of drug therapy amongst doctors and patients
- Changing attitudes and expectations on the part of doctors and patients with regard to health, including prevention and early treatment of potentially serious illness
- In particular, a generally more positive attitude to the healthcare of elderly people
- The continuing trend towards more and more treatment being provided in the community rather than in hospital—exemplified in shorter hospital stays and more care in the community for elderly people, mentally ill people and those with physical or learning disabilities.

Table 2.2 *Rise in net ingredient cost per prescription between 1982 and 1992*

	1982	**1992**	**% rise**
Children	£3.22	£4.42	37.3
Adults under pension age	£5.73	£7.53	31.4
Pensioners	£5.73	£6.70	16.9

Source: House of Commons Health Committee (1994)

the real price of existing (well-established) drugs had actually fallen by about a third, so that many drugs were cheaper for the NHS to buy, but the 'product mix' index, which is a measure of shift towards newer and relatively expensive preparations, had increased by an average of 5.5% in each year. The DoH described the product mix increase as being due to two factors—the doctor's propensity to prescribe recently introduced drugs rather than established ones, and the extent to which cost per prescription of new drugs reflects a premium over those of existing drugs (143% on average in recent years).

In summary, they calculated that between 1982 and 1992 the total NIC of drugs dispensed in the Family Health Service (FHS) rose by 60% in real terms.

Table 2.3 *Leading therapeutic groups (BNF chapters) by NIC (% of total NIC, £ million)*

BNF chapter	1982		1992		% rise 1992/1982
	NIC	%	NIC	%	
Cardiovascular	209.4	21.5	546.3	19.1	160.9
Central nervous system	140.4	14.4	307.7	10.8	119.2
Musculoskeletal and joint	118.5	12.2	231.2	8.1	95.1
Respiratory	97.9	10.1	342.2	12.0	249.5
Infections	93.9	9.7	203.0	7.1	116.2
Gastrointestinal	78.0	8.0	389.6	13.6	399.5
Skin	39.9	4.1	129.9	4.5	225.6
Endocrine	28.5	2.9	194.4	6.8	582.1
Obst/gyn, urinary tract	21.8	2.2	62.9	2.2	188.5
Nutrition and blood	16.2	1.7	82.9	2.9	411.7
ENT	12.0	1.2	35.1	1.2	192.5
Eye	10.2	1.1	39.1	1.4	283.3
Malignant disease and immunosuppression	8.9	0.9	71.8	2.5	706.7
Total (all chapters)	971.9	a	2858.0	a	194.1

Source: Health Committee, House of Commons, Second report 1993–4. Priority setting in the NHS: the NHS Drugs Budget. Volume II. Minutes of Evidence and Appendices. Replies from the Department of Health to Questions from the Health Committee (DB47).
[a] Percentage columns do not total 100% because not all BNF chapters are included in this table.
Crown Copyright, SDIE, DoH

This was the product of increases of
- 3% in 'pure demography'
- 27% in the number of prescriptions per head
- 11% in the average quantity of drugs per prescription
- 69% in the 'product mix' index,
- and incorporating a fall of 34% in the cost of existing drugs.

There have also been changes over the years in the kinds of drug prescribed. Table 2.3 shows changes in total net ingredient costs 1982–1992, without making any adjustment for inflation, which is not necessary for this comparison. The changes in net ingredient cost best reflect the factors described above, i.e. changes in volume and changes in the 'expensiveness' of drugs prescribed, mainly due to introduction of new drugs.

The rise in total NIC for all drugs over this period was 194%. In terms of this analysis, the most spectacular rise in share of overall costs has been for gastro-intestinal drugs, with a much smaller but significant rise for respiratory drugs. At the same time, the share of total costs occupied by other major groups (cardio-vascular, CNS, and musculoskeletal and joint) has decreased. The biggest rates of increase are, however, for the malignant disease and immunosuppression, endo-crine, and nutrition and blood chapters, where there have been important (but expensive) new advances in therapy and associated changes in medical practice.

For some therapeutic categories, the majority of prescriptions are for long-term treatment ('repeat prescriptions'). Once a patient is established on a satis-factory long-term therapy it is unlikely to be changed, so that some therapeutic groups may be more open to rapid changes in practice than others. For example,

Fig. 2.1 *Demographic pressure on prescribing expenditure (the average expenditure on drugs for elderly patients is up to 12 times greater than for younger patients). Source: Audit Commission (1994)*

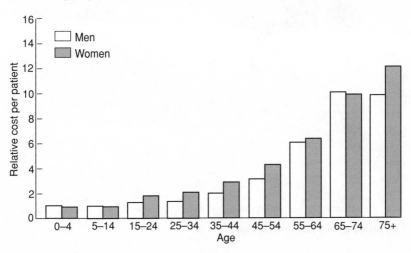

data from the Sowerby Foundation for Primary Care Informatics Research, Newcastle University, were used by the Audit Commission (Audit Commission, 1994) to show that the proportion of total costs accounted for by repeat pre-

Fig. 2.2 *Expenditure on prescribed drugs per prescribing unit (PU) adjusted for list inflation: 1992/93 (after adjustment for estimated list inflation, there was a 50% variation between the highest and the lowest spending FHSAs in average expenditure (net ingredient costs) on prescribed drugs per PU). Source: Audit Commission (1994)*

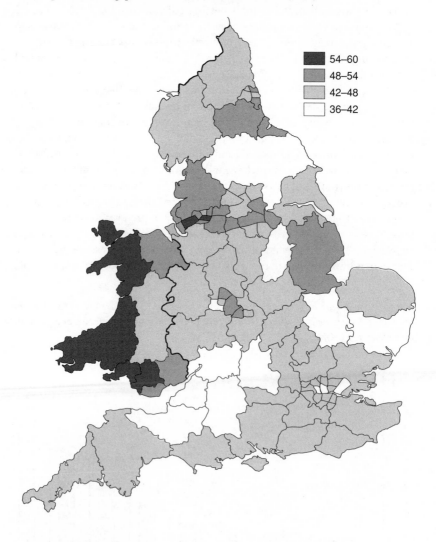

Note: The adjustment for list inflation assumes that it is spread evenly over patient age groups. No allowance has been made for variations in morbidity or need except for the age weighting included in the calculation of prescribing units.

scriptions varied from 25% for obstetric drugs and 30% for anti-infectives to 82% for gastrointestinal, 90% for respiratory, and 96% for cardiovascular drugs.

In the most comprehensive recent study of repeat prescribing in the UK, Harris and Dajda (1996) found that repeat prescriptions accounted for 75% of all items and 81% of costs and that more than 90% of prescriptions for patients aged over 85 were 'repeats'. A high proportion of general practice prescribing may therefore be relatively fixed and difficult to change, implying a recurrent liability well into the future (Fig. 2.1).

Medical practice variation

The fascination of prescribing data for research workers lies in the range of unexplained variation. At every level, from comparison of the prescribing of individual doctors or medical practices, through the comparison of regions to the comparison of nations, large differences in prescribing rates, whether by volume, cost, therapeutic group or individual drug, are characteristic of prescribing practice.

To be fair to prescribers, medical practice variation (MPV) is characteristic of most medical processes and procedures. For example, although it is common knowledge that operation rates for procedures such as hysterectomy and tonsillectomy vary markedly between countries (e.g. the USA and the UK), it is less well appreciated that they can vary to a marked extent within countries and within regions. Age and sex adjusted operation rates per 10 000 population in English regions have been shown to vary from 8.5 to 14.5 for hernias, 5.8 to 13.2 for prostatectomy, 18.1 to 28.7 for hysterectomy, 12.9 to 19.4 for appendectomy and 14.0 to 25.0 for tonsillectomy (House of Commons, Health Committee, 1994; Priority Setting in the NHS: Purchasing Table 4).

The variation is more to do with the kind of procedure than with national cultural differences or differences in medical systems, being greater for elective procedures (where there is a larger amount of discretion on the part of both patient and doctor) than for acute procedures such as appendectomy.

Similar variation can be shown in prescribing. Figure 2.2 shows a 50% variation in average expenditure (NIC per PU) between the highest and lowest spending FHSAs in England (1992/3). This is carried through into variation in prescribing frequency by therapeutic group (Table 2.4). If these differences were entirely due to justifiable demand, i.e. morbidity, the implied differentials in morbidity are large—twice as much respiratory disease in the North West as opposed to East Anglia, for example.

At the level of individual practices, however, and even within the same practice, there can be equally large variation in prescribing habits, suggesting that supply-side factors, that is the habits and attitudes of prescribers, are also important. Part of the answer is that, as with surgical procedures, most prescribing is elective and discretionary, with few instances where a medicine is absolutely essential (e.g. insulin).

Table 2.4 *Extremes of prescribing frequency by therapeutic group; English regions, number of prescriptions per 100 population per year*

	Lowest	Highest
Nervous system	98 (Oxford)	191 (North West)
Cardiovascular	85 (East Anglia)	156 (North West)
Respiratory	46 (East Anglia)	92 (North West)
Antirheumatic	30 (East Anglia)	48 (North West/Mersey))
Antibacterial	67 (East Anglia)	108 (North West)

Source: Department of Health (1989). *Health and personal social services statistics for England. HMSO, London.*

There is some evidence that the best pattern of prescribing might be described by low volume and high unit cost (Taylor, 1981) indicating parsimonious prescribing, but using drugs which are more expensive than average and, by implication, more modern and effective. Figure 2.4 shows how regions (e.g. Oxford) which have lower than average expenditure on medicines per NHS patient do tend to have higher average costs per prescription (although this is not quite the same as unit costs). Unit costs were analysed in a special study by Taylor (1981) which confirms this pattern (Table 2.5).

The argument about how far variation in prescribing is demand or supply led remains unresolved. Recent evidence has tended to emphasize that differences

Fig. 2.3 *Variation between GP practices in drug expenditure per prescribing unit: net ingredient costs 1992/93 (there are often marked differences between the prescribing of GP practices in the same locality. Low spending practices in high cost areas spend more than high spending practices in low cost areas).* ☐ *low cost FHSA with little list inflation;* ▨ *FHSA with highest average drug expenditure PU;—national all practices. Source: Audit Commission (1994)*

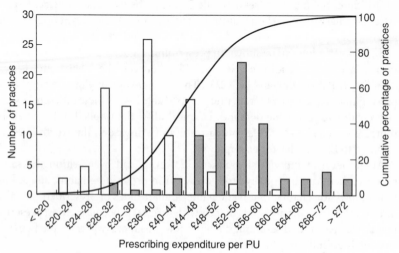

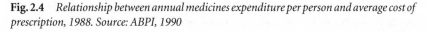

Fig. 2.4 *Relationship between annual medicines expenditure per person and average cost of prescription, 1988. Source: ABPI, 1990*

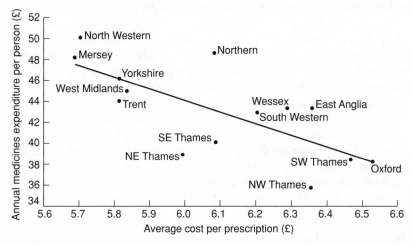

Table 2.5 *Cost and quality (Taylor 1981). Figures are illustrative proportional values in which the highest value is 100*

| | Low volume | | High volume | |
	High cost	Low cost	High cost	Low cost
[a]Index score	49	71	86	100
Repertory size	68	69	98	100
Recently introduced drugs	75	82	100	64
Cardiovascular	85	38	100	74
Cough/decongestant	55	58	100	64
Antibiotic	70	57	92	100

[a] Index of 'inappropriate' drugs

in demand (morbidity), even within small localities, may be much greater than previously thought.

At the level of individual practices, although Purves and Edwards (1993) found that the age–sex profile alone of a practice did not explain inter-practice variation in prescribing patterns, Healey *et al.* (1994) in a study of fundholding practices, showed that 97% of the variation in practice prescribing costs could be explained by differences in practice list size, the proportion of patients aged 65 years and over, the proportion of patients living in 'deprived areas' and whether or not the practice qualifies for 'inducement payments'.

At a higher level of aggregation of data, Family Health Services Authorities (FHSAs) in England and Wales, Forster and Frost (1991) found that 51% of the variation in prescription rates and 44% of the variation in prescribing costs could be explained by variation in age–sex structure. The standardized mortality ratio and the number of general practitioners per head of population, significantly improved the predictive power of their statistical model. Morton-Jones and Pringle (1993) found that two demographic factors (numbers of pensioners and the mobility of the registered population measured by list inflation) and two morbidity-related factors (standardized mortality ratios and numbers of prepayment certificates issued) explained 81% of the variation in NIC per registered patient between the 90 FHSAs in England and Wales.

There are, of course, well-established links between high mortality and low socio-economic status (Townsend *et al.*, 1988; Carstairs *et al.*, 1995). Pringle and Morton (1993) also found that prescribing in urban areas of northern England was characterized by high volume and low cost per item, whereas prescribing in southern semi-rural areas (generally more prosperous) was characterized by low volume and high cost per item. Unemployment rates were the most robust

Fig. 2.5 *Deprivation and health, Angina: prevalence by socio-economic status (rate per 1000) (Whitelaw et al., 1997)*

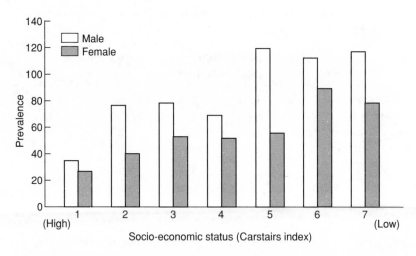

determinant of this inverse trend of number of items and cost per items. Lloyd *et al.* (1995) have shown that exemption from prescription charges on the grounds of poverty was a very significant marker of overall prescribing frequency in an area, whereas exemption on the grounds of being of pensionable age was not.

All of these studies used mortality rates and other indirect indicators of morbidity because, as mentioned earlier, direct morbidity data have hitherto been difficult to obtain. However, Figs 2.5 and 2.6 (Whitelaw *et al.*, 1997 in preparation) shows examples of marked socio-economic gradients in both morbidity

Fig. 2.6 *Deprivation and health, Nitrates: prescribing by socio-economic status (rate per 1000) (Whitelaw et al., 1997)*

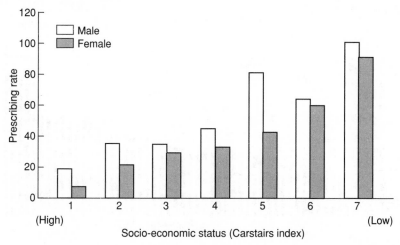

and prescribing found in a recent study of the health of 45–64 year olds in Scotland.

Increasing weight of evidence suggests that much MPV in prescribing may be related to differential morbidity associated with material deprivation. Nonetheless, there is plenty of evidence that prescribing is very far from standardized, despite the growth of local and practice formularies. Differences in the extent to

Fig. 2.7 *Variations in diagnosed morbidity between practices in one FHSA: percentage of patients identified as suffering from asthma (there are wide variations between neighbouring practices in the percentage of patients diagnosed as suffering from long-term chronic conditions). Source: Audit Commission (1994)*

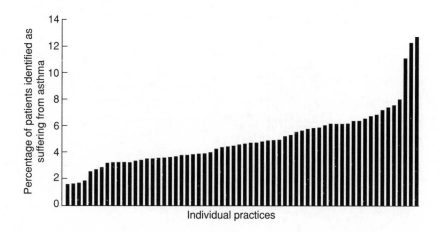

Fig. 2.8 *Variations in diagnosing morbidity between practices in one FHSA: percentage of patients identified as suffering from hypertension. Source: Audit Commission (1994)*

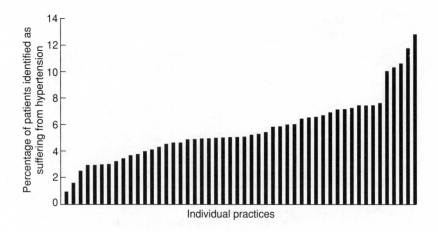

which genuine morbidity is identified and in how effectively it is treated might account for some inter-practice variation. In a study of 23 practices with low costs and 23 with high costs, McGavock (1988) found that, in high cost practices, half as many more patients with heart disease, asthma, diabetes and thyroid disease seemed to be treated than in practices with low costs. The Audit Commission report shows (Figs 2.7 and 2.8) the extent of variation between neighbouring practices in one FHSA in the percentages of patients identified as suffering from asthma and hypertension. Although there might be an element of

Fig. 2.9 *Variation in prescribing hypnotics and anxiolytics: number of days supply issued per prescribing unit (1992/93) (there is a wide variation in the extent to which drugs that can cause dependence at low doses are prescribed). Source: Audit Commission (1994)*

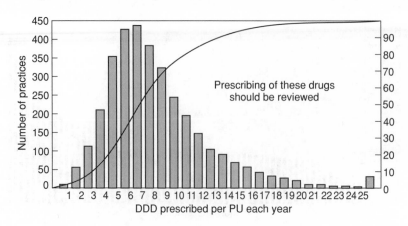

Fig. 2.10 *Drugs of limited clinical value: expenditure per prescribing unit (1992/93) (a saving of £45 million would be made if all doctors prescribed these drugs at similar rates per PU). Source: Audit Commission (1994)*

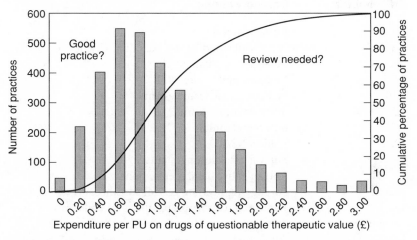

Expenditure per PU on drugs of questionable therapeutic value (£)

A national sample of 3,409 practices, selected to exclude those with atypical percentages of elderly patients.

overdiagnosis in some practices, these variations tend to suggest possible unidentified demand, rather than differences in readiness to prescribe.

Differences which are due more to the behaviour of the doctor than the patient are perhaps better examined by looking at the margins of prescribing—areas where prescribing is highly discretionary and/or where widespread prescribing of a particular drug or group of drugs is undesirable (Taylor, 1978). The Audit Commission examined prescribing of hypnotics and anxiolytics (Fig. 2.9) and of drugs which were considered to be of limited clinical value (Fig. 2.10 and Table 2.6) in a national sample of 3409 practices. Over England and Wales as a whole, the Audit Commission (1994) calculated that £45 millions (1.25% of the drug bill) could be saved by sensible reduction in the prescribing of these drugs.

McPherson (1994), in a discussion of MPV not related specifically to prescribing, distinguished three principle causes for systematic variation:

- clinical uncertainties
- ignorance of relevant research
- individual informed preferences.

The individual decision to prescribe for a particular patient can be separated from broader kinds of decision, made outwith the consulting room, about the range of drugs to be used (formularies) and the circumstances in which their use is appropriate (guidelines and decision support). The development of electronic on-screen systems of this kind (e.g. the *Electronic British National Formulary*, eBNF) and the *Prescribing RatiOnally with Decision Support In General*

Table 2.6 *Drugs of limited clinical value (Audit Commission, 1994, supported by comments from the British National Formulary)*

BNF chapter	Category of drug
1.4	Antidiarrhoeals
2.6.3	Peripheral vasodilators (excluding Thymoxamine)
2.6.4	Cerebral vasodilators
3.9.1	Cough suppressants
3.10	Systemic nasal decongestants
4.5	Appetite suppressants
9.7	Bitters and tonics
10.3.2	Topical NSAIDs
12.2.2	Topical nasal decongestants
12.2.3	Anti-infective nasal preparations
12.3.3	Lozenges, sprays and gels for sore throat
13.14	Topical circulatory preparations for chilblains

Practice Stud*Y*, PRODIGY) is likely to reduce MPV in prescribing, but 'evidence based medicine' is not a panacea, principally because there are so many gaps in the quantity and quality of evidence available to us. (Taylor, 1996)

McPherson (1994) acknowledged differences in the response of individual doctors because of differences in their experience, personalities, motivation and values, as well as in knowledge and skills:

Clinical knowledge may be perceived as collections of facts or truths, which comprise the dominant medical view. This can give rise to an awareness or anxiety that one knows only a small proportion of what can be known and may sometimes lead to lack of confidence and uncertainty, and this may result in some intellectual dishonesty. Today's medical facts may often be no more than current hypotheses, liable to be disproved and modified by new evidence.'

Subtle attitudinal differences were demonstrated in a study of over 200 GPs (Taylor and Bond, 1991). Doctors who showed favourable attitudes towards the pharmaceutical industry tended to be less concerned with the cost of drugs, more supportive of clinical independence, and more in favour of medicines (as opposed to other therapies) as a solution to patients' problems. They also showed a considerable variation in the size of 'repertories'—that is the number of different medicines each doctor prescribed—and similar variation in the rate at which doctors changed their repertories (Figs 2.11 and 2.13).

A purely 'medical' model does not fully explain the great complexity of the prescribing process. An elegant study by Howie (1976) demonstrated the effect of social factors on antibiotic prescribing and Harris (1980) identified four reasons for issuing prescriptions against his better pharmacological judgement:

Fig. 2.11 *Inter-relationship of attitudinal areas*

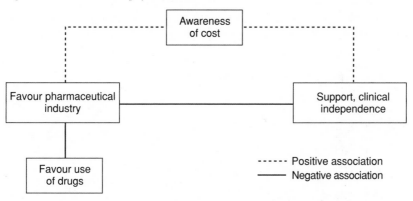

Fig. 2.12 *Size of doctors' repertoire*

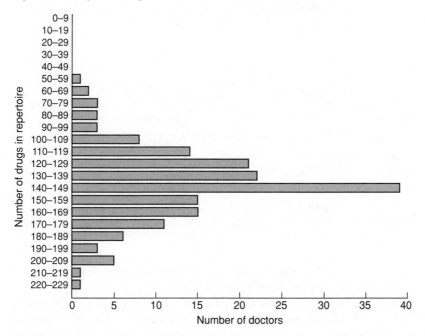

- the use of the prescription as a gift
- to maintain a relationship with the patient
- as a rejection—a way of getting rid of the patient
- as a response to some social need of the patient.

A study of 141 American physicians who were taking part in a trial of

Fig. 2.13 *Prescribing study: distribution of new items per 100 first items per doctor*

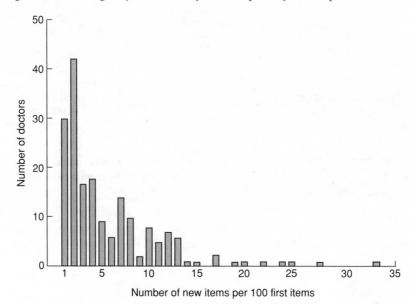

'academic detailing' (Schwartz *et al.*, 1989) also examined the motivations for their 'non-scientific' prescribing of drugs such as cerebral and peripheral vasodilators, propoxyphene and cephalexin (for upper respiratory infections). The most common reasons offered for use of these medications were:

- patient demand
- intentional use of the placebo effect
- own clinical experience not concordant with research evidence.

Pressure from patients is commonly claimed to be a major factor influencing doctors to prescribe unnecessarily or inappropriately, but Stimson (1976) showed that whereas doctors anticipated patients to expect a prescription in 80–90% of consultations, the actual expectation of patients for a prescription was much lower (30–50% of consultations). A more recent qualitative study (Britten, 1994) confirms that this is still the case.

In summary, it is likely that much MPV in prescribing can be explained by demand-side factors—differences in the volume and type of morbidity presented to the prescriber, in turn related particularly to socio-economic deprivation—but there remains an element of supply-side factors of the kind illustrated above. These factors are difficult to study, because they are likely to be related to differences in experience, personality, motivation and values, as well as knowledge and skills (McPherson, 1994). Although they may assume considerable importance in a minority of prescribers, it seems likely that they have a relatively small overall effect.

International comparisons

It might be expected that all of the factors which operate at national, regional and inter-doctor level also apply to international comparisons. For example, although evidence is scanty, it is thought that there are international differences in medicines usage which arise from national culture and upbringing. The large-scale use of traditional medicines in China and the extensive over the counter sales of 'tonic drinks' in Japan (Taido, 1994) are extreme examples but even within Western culture, where there is some sharing of tradition, dominant medical opinion may differ (e.g. in Germany low as well as high blood pressure is thought to require treatment) and in people's beliefs about their health. French doctors have high levels of prescribing for tranquillizers and vasodilators, whereas in Italy the use of these drugs has always been much more limited. In Italy, however, people are much more worried about their livers, leading to high sales of prescribed tonics and hepatic protectors (Taylor, 1992).

In a comparison of prescribing in Italy, France, Germany and the UK, Garratini (1995) found that, of the 50 most heavily sold products, only seven active principles were common to the four countries. In Germany use of fixed ratio combinations of reserpine and diuretics persisted as the leading treatment for hypertension long after their use had virtually disappeared in the UK and Sweden, and there were also major differences in use of cardiac glycosides (Gross, 1984). Sunol *et al.* (1991) reported that the number of registered pharmaceutical specialties was 21 000 in Germany (2900 active substances) and 1000 (700) in Iceland. Thiazide consumption in Sweden was 10 times that of Spain, in DDDs per head of population. These variations are, of course, not entirely due to variation in prescribing by GPs. Guglielmo *et al.* (1994) found great variation in the use of antimicrobial drugs in hospitals, both between countries, within the same country and between patients with the same infectious disease.

It is likely that there are also genuine international differences in demand, due to differential morbidity and differential identification of morbidity which are, in part, a function of differing systems of medical care (Table 2.7).

However, in making international, as opposed to intra-UK, comparisons, the influences of governments and healthcare systems obviously assume greater importance. Most EU governments which operate state-supported health systems like the UK face a dilemma which, broadly expressed, is the tension between promoting a healthy pharmaceutical industry (good for the economy) and economic prescribing (good for the individual and the health service). Most have mechanisms for regulating drug prices, through controls on manufacturers, and/or regulating patient demand, through prescription charges of some kind. The price of the same drug in different countries can vary enormously. For example, at one time Zyloric was 10 times more expensive in the UK than in Spain, Indocid was 10 times more expensive in the Netherlands than in Greece, and Microgynon was 8 times more expensive in Germany than in France (Taylor, 1992).

In general, I believe the UK has managed to strike a good balance between the competing interests of the Department of Trade and the Department of Health (Fig. 2.14).

Differential activity of the pharmaceutical industry and differential regulation of its promotional activities may be another factor in international variations in drug use. The UK's rules in this respect are fairly tight, limiting promotional expenditure to about 10% of sales as opposed to 15–20% in other

Table 2.7 *Internation comparison of rates for premature (<69 years) death from coronary heart disease (CHD) and stroke in men and women. Age-standardized mortality rates (per 100000) (Uemura and Pisa, 1988)*

Country	CHD Men	CHD Women	Stroke Men	Stroke Women
N. Ireland	406	130	62	50
Scotland	398	142	73	57
Finland	390	79	74	43
Czechoslovakia	346	101	130	75
England and Wales	318	94	52	40
New Zealand	296	94	46	38
Australia	247	76	44	33
USA	235	80	34	26
Poland	230	54	72	47
Greece	135	33	60	44
Portugal	104	32	20	74
France	94	20	45	21
Japan	38	13	79	45

European countries. The ratio of pharmaceutical company representatives to population is also lower in the UK than in many other European countries (Table 2.8).

Table 2.8 *Number of pharmaceutical company representative per head of population in various European countries (Orton, Fry, 1995)*

Country	No. of representatives	Rate per head of population
UK	6000	1 : 9667
Spain	9000	1 : 4333
Germany	15000	1 : 4000
France	15000	1 : 3800
Italy	17000	1 : 3412

In an international survey of sources of information about new drugs and atti-

Fig. 2.14 *Price level of a 'basket' of 125 drugs. Index (cheapest country = 100). (De Smedt, 1992)*

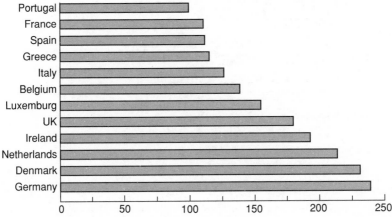

tudes towards prescribing, Hull and Marshall (1987) found major disagreement amongst primary care physicians about the importance of information from drug company representatives. For example, in Sweden and Yugoslavia representatives were highly rated as a source of information about new drugs, whereas in the UK and Belgium they were poorly rated. Such differences may partly explain why UK doctors are relatively conservative in their uptake of new medicines (Fig. 2.15).

A frequently quoted Italian study (Garattini and Garattini, 1993) also showed that UK doctors compared extremely favourably with those in other European countries in their choice of good, effective 'first line' drugs as opposed to 'second line' and 'ineffective drugs' (Table 2.9).

Because of differences in the division between prescribed and non-prescribed drugs the best international comparisons are probably of total drug utilization. In general, the more wealthy a country, the more it spends on healthcare, and on medicines, whether prescribed or non-prescribed.

Table 2.9 *Pharmaceutical prescriptions in four European countries: the 50 most widely sold products in efficacy-related categories (Garratini and Garratini, 1993)*

Country	Rating A	B	C
Italy	25	15	10
France	26	14	10
Germany	35	9	6
UK	45	4	0

A, drugs with proven efficacy from RCT evidence.

B, second line drugs and combinations.

C, no evidence of efficacy.

Fig. 2.15 *1987 sales of all products introduced in the previous five years as a share of total 1987 sales. Source: ABPI*

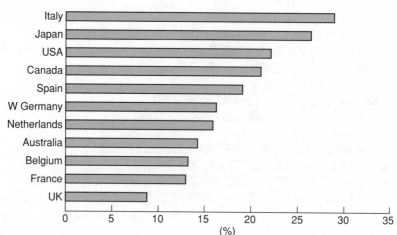

In terms of total (private and public) spending on all healthcare, the UK position is modest (Fig. 2.16) and it is particularly interesting that USA public expenditure on healthcare is similar to UK: i.e. USA spends as much on its limited public system of healthcare as UK does on the whole of the NHS.

In terms of spending on medicines the UK position is also conservative, even although OTC sales are greater here than in some other European countries (Fig. 2.17).

In conclusion, therefore, although there is no reason to be complacent, international comparisons suggest that UK prescribers are relatively conservative and effective in their choice of drugs and that overall medicines consumption in the UK is relatively modest. This position may be threatened by a number of impending changes. These are mainly to do with the vast power of an increasingly globalized pharmaceutical industry.

Some elements of industry see the UK as an underexploited market for medicines (Memorandum submitted by the American Pharmaceutical Group. In House of Commons Health Committee, 1994); increasing deregulation (from prescription only to pharmacy status) is likely to increase overall medicines consumption (see also Chapter 10); and finally, the creation of a European Medicines Evaluation Agency will reduce the importance of national institutions such as the UK Committee on Safety of Medicines, and might make it easier for powerful industrial and allied interests to dominate regulatory activities in the EC (Taylor, 1992).

Comparison of public and private expenditure on healthcare.

Fig. 2.16 *Expenditure on health (% GDP) (Goss, 1993)*

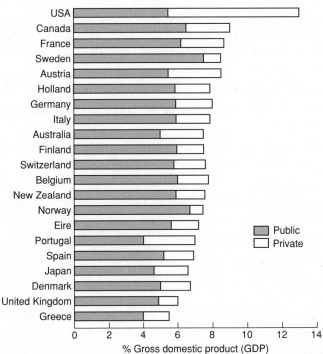

Fig. 2.17 *International comparisons: pharmaceutical expenditure per person.*
Source: Audit Commission, 1994

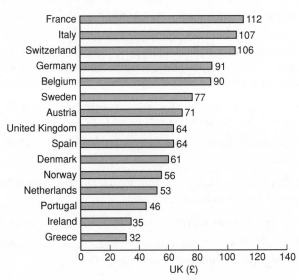

References

American Pharmaceutical Group Memorandum (1994). In House of Commons Health Committee (1994). *Second Report Session 1993–4. Priority setting in the NHS: the NHS drugs budget. Volume II: Minutes of evidence and appendices.* HMSO, London.

Anis, A. H., Carruthers, S. G., Carter, A. O., Keirulf, J. (1996). Variability in prescription drug utilization: issues for research. *Canadian Medical Journal,* **154**(5), 635–40.

APBI (1990). *Pharmaceutical Briefing 10.* Association of the British Pharmaceutical Industry, London.

Audit Commission (1994). *A prescription for improvement: towards more rational prescribing in general practice.* HMSO, London.

Boydell, L., Grandidier, H., Rafferty, C., McAteer, C., Reilly, P. (1995). General practice data retrieval: the Northern Ireland Project. *Journal of Epidemiology and Community Health,* **49** (Suppl. 1), 22–5.

Britten, N. (1994). Patient demand for prescriptions: a view from the other side. *Family Practice,* **11**, 62–6.

Carstairs, V., Morris, R. (1991). *Deprivation and health in Scotland.* Aberdeen University Press, Aberdeen.

Department of Health (1989). *Health and personal social services statistics for England.* HMSO, London.

DeSmedt, M. (1992). International comparison of drug prices. In *Drug utilization studies: Report of the WHO Drug Utilization Research Group.* WHO Regional Office for Europe, Copenhagen.

Fleming, D. M., Fullarton, J. (1993). *The application of a general practice database to pharmaco epidemiology.* Occasional Paper No. 62. London: Royal College of General Practitioners.

Forster, D. P., Frost, C. E. (1991). Use of regression analysis to explain the variation in prescribing rates and costs between family practitioner committees. *British Journal of General Practice,* **41**, 67–71.

Garattini, S. (1995). Pharmaceutical prescriptions in Italy. *International Journal of Technology Assessment in Health Care,* **11**(3), 417–27.

Garattini, S., Garattini, L. (1993). Pharmaceutical prescriptions in four European countries. *Lancet,* **342**: 1191–2.

Gilleghan, J. D. (1991). *Prescribing in general practice.* Occasional Paper No. 54, Royal College of General Practitioners, London.

Goss, B. (1993). You are all my patients. In *Rationing in action.* BMJ Publishing, London.

Gross, F. H. (1984). Drug utilization data in risk/benefit analyses of drugs—benefit analysis. *Acta Medica Scandinavica—Supplementum,* **683**, 141–7.

Guglielmo, L., Leone, R., Moretti, U., Conforti, A., Velo, G. P. (1994). Antimicrobial drug utilization in Italy and other European countries [Review]. *Infection*, **22**, Suppl. 3, S176–81.

Harris, C., Dajda, R. (1996). The scale of repeat prescribing. *British Journal of General Practice*, **412**, 649–53.

Harris, C. M. (1980). Personal view. *British Medical Journal*, **2**, 57.

Healey, A. T., Yule, B. F., Reid, J. P. (1994). Variations in general practice prescribing costs and implications for budget setting. *Health Economics*, **3**(1), 47–56.

House of Commons Health Committee (1995). *First report, session 1994–5. Priority Setting in the NHS: Purchasing. Volume I.* HMSO, London.

House of Commons Health Committee (1994). *Second report, session 1993–4. Priority setting in the NHS: the NHS drugs budget. Volume II: minutes of evidence and appendices.* HMSO, London.

Howie, J. G. R. (1976). Clinical judgement and antibiotic use in general practice. *British Medical Journal*, **2**, 1061–4.

Hull, F. M., Marshall, T. (1987). Sources of information about new drugs and attitudes towards drug prescribing: an international study of differences between primary care physicians. *Family Practice*, **4**(2), 123–8.

Jick, H., Jick, S., Derby, L. (1991). Validation of information on general practitioner computerized data resource in the United Kingdom. *British Medical Journal*, **302**, 766–8.

Jick, H., Terris, B. Z., Derby, L. E., Jick, S. S. (1992). Further validation of information recorded on general practitioner based computerized data resource in the United Kingdom. *Pharmacoepidemiology and Drug Safety*, **1**, 347–9.

Lee, D., Bergman, U. (1989). Studies of drug utilization. In *Pharmacoepidemiology*, ed. B. L. Strom. Churchill Livingstone, New York.

Lloyd, D. C., Harris, C. M., Clucas, D.W. (1995). Low income scheme index (LISI): a new deprivation scale based on prescribing in general practice. *British Medical Journal*, **310**, 165–9.

McGavock, H. (1988). Some patterns of prescribing by urban general practitioners. *British Medical Journal*, **296**, 900–2.

McPherson, K. (1994). How should health policy be modified by the evidence of medical practice variations? In *Controversies in health care policies*, ed. M. Marinker. BMJ Publishing, London.

Morton-Jones, T., Pringle, M. (1993). Explaining variations in prescribing costs across England. *British Medical Journal*, **306**, 1731–4.

Orton, P., Fry, J. (1995). *UK health care: The facts.* Kluwer Academic Publishers, Dordrecht, Netherlands.

Pringle, M., Morton-Jones, A. (1994). Using unemployment rates to predict prescribing trends in England. *British Journal of General Practice*, **44**, 53–6.

Purves, I. N., Edwards, C. (1993). Comparison of prescribing unit with index including both age and sex in assessing general practice prescribing costs. *British Medical Journal*, **306**, 496–8.

Schwartz, R. K., Soumerai, S. B., Avorn, J. (1989). Physician motivations for nonscientific prescribing. *Social Science and Medicine*, **28(6)**, 577–82.

Stimson, G. V. (1976). In Prescribing in General Practice. *Journal of the Royal College of General Practitioners*, **26** (Suppl. 1), 88–96.

Strom, B. L. (ed.) (1989). *Pharmacoepidemiology*. Churchill Livingstone, New York.

Sunol, R., Abello, C., Cels, I. C. (1991). Studies in utilization of drugs: a review of different methods. *Quality Assurance in Health Care*, **3**(1), 63–72.

Taido, N. (1994). The role of tonic drinks in the Japanese OTC market. *Pharmacology (Basel)* **16**(11S): 38–42.

Taylor, D. (1992). Prescribing in Europe—forces for change. In *Medicine in Europe*, ed. T. Richards. BMJ Publishing, London. .

Taylor, M. W., Ritchie, L. D., Taylor, R. J., Ryan, M. P., Paterson, N. I. A., Duncan, R., Brotherston, K. G. (1990). General practice computing in Scotland. *British Medical Journal*, **300**, 170–2.

Taylor, R. J. (1978). Prescribing costs and patterns of prescribing in general practice. *Journal of the Royal College of General Practitioners*, **28**, 531–5.

Taylor, R. J. (1981). General practice prescribing in North East Scotland. MD Thesis, University of Aberdeen. (Relevant section briefly described in Gilleghan (1991)).

Taylor, R. J. (1996). Experts and evidence. *British Journal of General Practice*, **46**, 268–70.

Taylor, R. J., Bond, C. M. (1991). Change in the established prescribing habits of general practitioners: an analysis of initial prescriptions in general practice. *British Journal of General Practice*, **41**, 244–8. [Further unpublished details on attitudinal studies are available from the author.]

Tomson, G. (1991). Drug utilization studies and people. A Swedish perspective. [Review.] *Annali dell Instituto Superiore di Sanita*, **27**(2): 239–45.

Townsend, P., Davidson, N., Whitehead, M. (eds) (1988). *Inequalities in health: the Black report and the health divide*. Penguin, London.

Uemura, K., Pisa, Z. (1988). Trends in cardiovascular disease mortality in industrialized countries since 1950. *World Health Statistics Quarterly*, **41**(3/4), 155–78.

Whitelaw, F. G., Taylor, R. J., Nevin, S. L., Taylor, M. W., Milne, R. M., Watt, A. H. (1996). Completeness and accuracy of morbidity and repeat prescribing records held on general practice computers in Scotland. *British Journal of General Practice*, **46**, 181–6.

Whitelaw, F. G., Taylor, R. J., Nevin, S. L., Watt, A. H. (1997). Deprivation and health: associations between morbidity, repeat prescribing and socio-economic status in the middle aged population of Scotland. In preparation.

Further reading

Avorn, J., Chen, M., Hartley, R. (1982). Scientific versus commercial sources of influence on the prescribing behaviour of physicians. *American Journal of Medicine*, **73**(1), 4–8.

Anon, (1994). European Medicines Evaluation Agency and the new licensing arrangements. *Drug and Therapeutics Bulletin*, **32**, 89–90.

Benzeval, M., Judge, K., Whitehead, M. (eds.) (1995). *Tackling inequalities in health: an agenda for action.* King's Fund, London.

Bergman, U. (1989). Pharmaco-epidemiological prespectives [Review]. *Pharmaceutisch Weekblad—Scientific Edition*, **11**(5), 151–4.

Bradley, C. P. (1991). Decision making and prescribing patterns—a literature review. *Family Practice*, **8**, 276–87.

Department of Health (1994). Replies from the Department of Health to Questions from the Health Committee. Health Committee, House of Commons, *Second report 1993–4. Priority setting in the NHS: the NHS drugs budget. Volume II: Minutes of evidence and appendices* (DB47).

Ryan, M. P. (1989). A system for general practice computing in Scotland. *Health Bulletin (Edinburgh)* **47**, 110–19.

Serradell, J., Bjornson, D. C., Hartzema, A. G. (1987). Drug utilization study methodologies: national and international perspectives. *Drug Intelligence and Clinical Pharmacy*, **21**(12), 994–1001.

Sleator, D. J. D. (1993). Towards accurate prescribing analysis in general practice: accounting for the effects of practice demography. *British Journal of General Practice*, **43**, 102–6.

CHAPTER THREE

The development of new drugs

Richard Hobbs and David Millson

The main objectives of clinical novel therapeutic research are to demonstrate the efficacy, safety, and metabolism of a drug or device in defined clinical indications, with the dosage range and proposed market formulation defined, and culminating in a successful approval from drug regulatory authorities. More recently, there has been a greater expectation that novel drugs will demonstrate efficacy over and above that seen in existing therapies and also provide some evidence on cost-effectiveness. Most new drugs are developed exclusively within the pharmaceutical industry, although academic medicine can sometimes play a role in the initial generation of new clinical entities or the hypothesis of new clinical indications for existing therapies.

The development of new drugs is a costly, high risk, resource intensive venture where the odds of overall success with a new chemical entity (NCE) entering clinical trials are greater than 30 to 1. A new drug discovery programme may take 3–5 years to produce a candidate drug and a further 5 years to complete clinical trials, before launch as a successful product. The later a problem arises during development the greater the investment lost if development is stopped.

Withdrawal of a drug early, particularly before clinical trials have started, incurs relatively little penalty. Termination of a project just before licensing approval may result in development costs exceeding £100 million. During later development, about 30% of projects are terminated because of lack of efficacy, and a further 30% because of unfavourable pharmacokinetics and metabolism (e.g. short half-life, incomplete and variable absorption, enzyme induction, or high first-pass elimination). Of the remaining 30%, 1 in 4 is stopped for commercial reasons. The net result is that a very small proportion of candidate products eventually reach the market.

The future pharmaceutical market is likely to consist of only a few key organizations of a certain critical mass, hence the recent wave of mergers and takeovers, such as Smith Kline Beecham, Bristol Myers Squibb, and Glaxo-Wellcome. However, despite its size, a pharmaceutical giant like Glaxo-Wellcome, which employs over 58000 people world-wide, is worth over £20 billion and has annual profits approaching £3 billion, commands only 5% of the world drug market with the remaining 20–30 top companies each accounting for 1–5% of sales (Gustafsson *et al.*, 1992; Arendt, 1995).

Many companies owe their success to 'blockbuster' drugs, for which yearly sales and profits often exceed £1 billion. Successful companies try to overcome dependence on a single drug by diversifying their portfolio, spreading the risk of success or failure across a number of products.

Pre-trials research

The impetus to develop new clinical entities has evolved with the increasing complexity of the processes needed to develop new drugs. Early compounds were often developed in response to observation of the clinical effects of ingesting natural products. Examples of currently used drugs that were isolated from 'natural experimentation' are digoxin, morphine, and aspirin. All of these compounds were isolated as active ingredients in traditional remedies.

A further impetus to develop new drugs is the potential therapeutic impact of the new compound or the scale of the likely market. Compounds that are effective in otherwise life-threatening or fatal illnesses will therefore have an immediate place in management. One example of this was the development of insulin for insulin-dependent diabetics, previously a fatal illness with a relatively short prognosis. In contrast, drugs which are effective at symptom control may be worth developing, even if they have no influence over disease progression, assuming the prevalence of illness is high. Compounds active in pain control of arthritic disease, such as non-steroidal anti-inflammatories (NSAIDs) and analgesics, therefore have considerable potential. Indeed, if disease prevalence is high (a reflection of incidence of disease and length of prognosis), then this is likely to stimulate development of a high number of different clinical entities active within that defined therapeutic area. Such drug development may even produce a range of compounds with similar modes of action, the so-called 'me too' drugs.

Pre-trials research: *in vitro* and animal studies

Having identified the potential need for an NCE, then the first step in drug development is to synthesize active substances, in other words chemicals which will have the biological effects intended. This can be a laborious process, with perhaps 10000 molecules being screened as potential new products, but further laboratory testing identifying only a few compounds (perhaps only 10–15 of the 10000 screened) that seem worthy of further investigation. The increasing use of computers in drug development is likely to produce some shortcuts: use of molecular modelling and a much better understanding of the action of drugs at a molecular level can aid the prediction of likely effects, and even adverse effects, of new molecules.

Having produced these new chemicals to test, early investigations will then involve *in vitro* testing against banks of compounds for whom their effects are well documented. This will produce data upon the likely action of the NCE and help define its likely area of activity. The full chemical requirements for an NCE are summarized in Box 3.1.

Box 3.1 *Chemical and pharmaceutical requirements of an NCE*

Chemical structure
Potential isomerism
Physicochemical properties (solubility, polymorphism, pK_a, pH, etc.)
Analytical specification (impurities)
Stability testing
Sterility testing
Pyrogen testing
Storage conditions

For compounds that look promising, it is now also possible to do more *in vitro* studies of drugs on living cells, tissues, or organs that provide additional information on potential action. This aspect of drug development has been extremely important at reducing the numbers of animals needed to test for drug efficacy and safety, since as much research as possible will be done on compounds *in vitro*. However, it is unlikely that we will ever reach the stage that no drug testing is required in animals at all, since it is likely that whatever the sophistication of computer modelling and *in vitro* testing, there will be a desire to replicate this data in live animals prior to exposure to human volunteers.

This area of drug development will rightly remain an extremely sensitive issue and there will continue to be exploration of ways of reducing the numbers of animals needed for clinical research. Indeed, one important benefit from changes in the regulation of drug developments at a national and international level is that greater conformity between countries on the evidence that needs to be provided for regulatory purposes will reduce the number of animals needed for experimentation.

The current role of animal studies is therefore to confirm:
- mode of action of the compound
- efficacy of effect
- pharmokinetics (absorption and excretion)
- acute toxicology (see Table 3.1)
- chronic tolerance of the compound (at least 6 months' dosing)
- toxicology on genetic component of cells
- toxicology on fetal development.

Table 3.1 *Requirements for duration of toxicity studies*

Duration of toxicity studies in animals	Intended duration of dosing in humans
EU requirements	
14 days	Single dose or several doses on 1 day
28 days	Repeated up to 7 days
90 days	Repeated up to 30 days
180 days	Repeated beyond 30 days
Nordic country requirements	
14 days	Single dose to few people
28 days	Repeated for 1–2 weeks
90 days	Repeated for 1–3 months
180 days to 2 years	Repeated for 6 months or more
US requirements (Phases I and II)	
14 days	1–3 days
28 days	Up to 4 weeks
90 days	Longer than 4 weeks

In Canada, 12 months' toxicity studies in animals are required where dosing in humans exceeds 1 month

The final important need for animal studies is to help determine suitable dosages of promising compounds for use in human volunteer studies. Although there are considerable differences between animal species, such as physiological response to drugs or their metabolism, the information provided from such trials provides crucial data on minimizing the risk to humans at the point an application is made for permission to commence human clinical trials (see Box 3.2). In the UK this involves an application to the Committee on Safety of Medicines for a Clinical Trials Certificate (CTC).

Box 3.2 *Preclinical data needed before administering an NCE to humans*

Mutagenicity screening tests
Animal toxicology
Safety pharmacology
Whole body autoradiography (labelled drug required)
Pharmacokinetic and metabolic studies in animals (specific assay required)

Pre-trials research: the target product profile

Before embarking on a drug development programme, a target product profile (TPP) is produced. The TPP is a projection at least 5 years into the future, setting out the minimum requirements which will make the new medicine successful in the highly competitive pharmaceutical marketplace. Constructing the TPP requires market intelligence from many available sources (scientific meetings, publications, clinical advisory mechanisms, and the market research) combined with medical and scientific knowledge based on the following criteria:

- **Disease incidence, prevalence and epidemiology**. For example malaria, sickle cell disease and other 'tropical diseases' are exceedingly common on a world-wide basis, but are not likely to become the targets of drug discovery programmes because of problems of healthcare delivery and the lack of return on investment from the principal pharmaceutical markets.
- **Perceived benefits of a pioneer therapy**. Attempts to produce a more effective antiplatelet agent than aspirin after myocardial infarction are thwarted by the difficulties of showing an incremental clinical benefit over aspirin, except in trials involving tens of thousands of patients. (Sandercock *et al.*, 1994), which would have little chance of demonstrating a cost-effective alternative that would pay back the costs of research and development.
- **Technical feasibility and pharmacological innovativeness**. Melatonin and melatonin agonists provide a an attractive treatment for jet lag, but would be difficult to exploit commercially because of the public information disclosure, with little opportunity to introduce a novel drug with adequate intellectual property protection and with a price premium relative to melatonin.
- **Patentability of treatment concept and chemical synthesis**. Whole segments of human gene sequences are covered by patents, which could preclude the development of clinical diagnostic kits for gene disorders or might hinder focused drug discovery of gene targets.
- **Commercial viability considers overall costs of manufacture and development, marketing in relation to peak sales**. Many monoclonal antibody 'biotech' products require low-yield expensive fermentation facilities where the cost of production potentially exceeds the marketing cost of the drug.

Therefore, in developing any drug the opportunity cost of capital used has to be balanced against the risk and return on investment which could be achieved by altering the priorities and therapeutic balance of a portfolio.

Most pharmaceutical companies rely on shareholder investment to support research and have to expose themselves to market analysts at 'show and tell' meetings where they have to justify their research strategy.

Box 3.3 provides a hypothetical example of a TPP relating to a new class of antihypertensive agent called Losentin which will act by blocking the elevated levels of the pressor substance angiotensin II which occurs in hypertensive subjects. The decision to embark on a research programme can be seen to relate to the research skills base of a pharmaceutical company together with an overall

41

Fig. 3.1 *Relative directional policy matrix scores for an 'ideal' drug and for Losentin 1st and 2nd to the market*

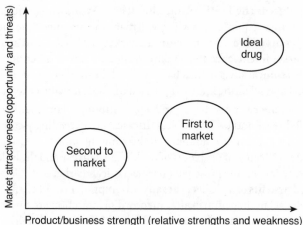

risk:benefit analysis. During this critical phase external consultation with academic experts and groups of medical practitioners will be sought.

GPs may be approached to seek their opinion of the likely merits of a potential new therapy based on the TPP. This intelligence gathering is likely to involve either a structured interview or questionnaire which will try to determine:

• Does the GP actively treat the target patient population or is treatment more often initiated as a result of a specialist hospital consultation?
• Is the condition common in general practice, is it acute or chronic, do patients seek treatment or do they rely on self-medication?
• What current therapy is available for the condition in general practice and how satisfied are both patient and doctor with it?
• Are there any unmet medical needs and to what extent could these be met by the perceived new therapy as outlined in the target product profile?
• How close to ideal is the TPP?

Pharmaceutical companies then score elements within the TPP and apply decision analysis techniques, which allow comparisons to be made across a whole research portfolio. Thus the relatively low technical but high commercial risk of developing a new antihypertensive treatment can be compared with the high technical risk but highly favourable commercial potential of an effective treatment for dementia.

Figure 3.1 shows a hypothetical decision policy matrix for Losentin and demonstrates the critical importance of being first to the market with the 'ideal drug' occupying a place in the far right corner of the matrix.

Box 3.3   *TPP for the hypothetical drug Losentin*

Clinical indication

'Losentin' is a once daily orally active angiotensin II antagonist which is indicated for the treatment of moderate to severe hypertension.

Essential attributes

- once daily oral dosing to aid compliance
- effective as monotherapy with a fixed dose regimen
- well tolerated in the elderly and in special patient risk groups (i.e. patients with hepatic and renal impairment or diabetics)
- first or second product to reach market place
- no potential for adverse drug interactions or incompatibility with commonly used antihypertensives.

Scientific and technical feasibility

The angiotensin type I receptor and cellular transduction mechanism are well characterized. Furthermore, animal and clinical models, such as antagonism of intravenous angiotensin II induced hypertension can be used as surrogate endpoints to predict efficacy and likely duration of effects in humans—*therefore development of Losentin has low technical risk.*

Commercial and marketing assessment

At least three candidate drugs are in late phase clinical evaluation (phase II–I). Unless an NCE shows longer duration of action (i.e. once daily dosing) or improved clinical properties leading to increased market penetration, the net product value will be low (<£50M)—*therefore development of Losentin has high commercial risk.*

Scope of clinical and regulatory programme

FDA and other regulatory guidelines exist which clearly define the development path required to achieve a successful registration for an novel antihypertensive agent. In excess of 4000 patients will be studied. Expensive long-term animal oncogenicity and toxicity will be required, together with long term follow-up in patients. *Therefore, clinical and regulatory risks for Losentin are low but development costs are high.*

Phases of drug development in humans

In this section the different phases of drug development in humans will be discussed, highlighting the potential involvement and issues arising which might

Fig. 3.2 *Discovery and development of a new medicine: stages and timescales*

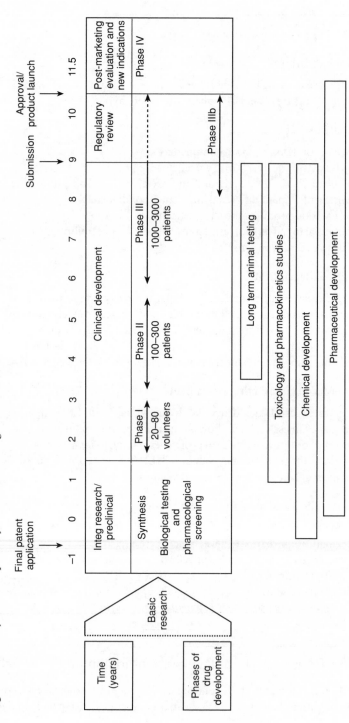

affect the GP either as an active participant, an interested bystander, or a final customer of the marketed pharmaceutical product. At each stage examples of ethical, scientific and clinical dilemmas will be considered and practical advice offered from a primary care perspective.

Drug development is classically divided into phases I–IV (see Fig. 3.2 for flow diagram showing stages and time scale for development of medicines).

Phases I and II: the exploratory or concept testing trials

The main functions of early studies with an NCE in humans are summarized in Box 3.4. For most drugs phase I trials will be initiated in healthy volunteers, often in a purpose-built clinical pharmacology unit equipped to a high standard with the latest resuscitation and monitoring equipment. Studies will be carried out under the supervision of a physician with a special interest in monitoring the pharmacological activity of the NCE and relating its effects to the plasma concentration profile or pharmacokinetics. Increasingly clinical research organizations (CROs) are responsible for the conduct of these studies. CROs are sometimes attached to academic centres or in partnership with a healthcare trust, but more usually operate in the commercial sector.

Box 3.4 *The purpose of early studies with an NCE in humans*

To answer two important questions:

- Is the drug likely to be safe and well tolerated?
- Is the specified pharmacological effect seen in animals also seen in humans?

To obtain pharmacokinetic and metabolic data

The main objectives of phase I studies are to:
- assess safety and tolerability against the predicted animal pharmacology and toxicology
- investigate the relationship between plasma or tissue concentration and the desirable pharmacological effect (e.g. blood pressure lowering)
- describe the dose response and range of useful doses, avoiding unnecessary toxicity
- choose a surrogate endpoint which will aid dose ranging and with predictive value in patients with deranged target pathology (e.g. enzyme inhibition or receptor blockade).

Often phase I studies may involve a provocation challenge. For example, the dermal flare response to intradermal serotonin for 5-HT3 receptor antagonists has been used to determine the clinically useful dose and duration of effect for the 5-HT3 receptor antagonist Alosetron (Millson *et al.*, 1992) (see Fig. 3.3). Another strategy is to will employ a disease model, such as the ipecacuanha emesis model in healthy volunteers to predict the antiemetic potency of ondansetron (Minton, 1994) (see Fig. 3.4), for concept testing before exposing larger numbers of patients in clinical trials to potentially toxic or sub-therapeutic doses of an NCE.

Fig. 3.3 *Dermal flare response to 5-HT3 receptor antagonist to determine dose and duration response (Millson et al. 1992)*

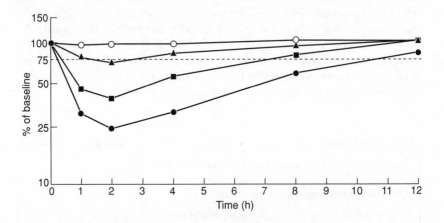

Because phase I studies are carried out on healthy volunteers they are 'risk only' studies where the altruistic or financial motive of the volunteer must be balanced against the 'greater good' and prospect of a new therapy which might benefit humanity as a whole.

Setting aside the ethical dilemma as to whether drug testing should be conducted on patients who might stand to benefit, rather than on healthy non-patient volunteers studies, conducting phase I studies in healthy volunteers has a number of potential advantages:

• less physiological variation and more uniform pharmacological responses
• more stamina and ability to comply with complex and time-consuming experimental paradigms
• no clinical problems associated with stopping effective treatments or administering inadequate doses or placebo
• possibility of cross-over designs giving more statistical power with fewer subjects.

GPs may be involved in the conduct of such trials in a limited capacity by

Fig. 3.4 *Probability of prevention by ondansetron of ipecacuanha-induced emesis in healthy volunteers. Each data point represents the percentage of a each group of ten volunteers not experiencing emesis. Estimated ED50 for protection against emesis: 1.27 mg (standard error 0.29 mg, correlation coefficient 0.867). (From Minton, 1994)*

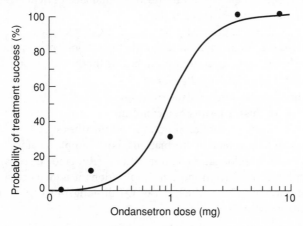

providing the medical review of research protocols as a member or an ethical review body, or by providing important background confidential medical information on a patient who wishes to become a 'healthy volunteer'. It is important to realize that for phase I trials carried out in the UK, pharmaceutical companies are self-regulated and are currently not required to consult with or obtain regulatory permission to conduct studies in healthy volunteers. With the exception of a small number of moderately severe (0.55%) and even fewer (0.04%) potentially life threatening or fatal adverse events reported in a large (>8100 subjects) confidential survey (Orme *et al.*, 1989), phase I studies in the UK are considered to be adequately covered by current arrangements and to carry an acceptable risk to volunteers.

A GP who accepts an invitation to sit on an ethical review committee may wish to consider the research guidelines of the Royal College of Physicians, the Medical Research Council, and the British Pharmaceutical Industry (ABPI). The important considerations to be addressed by ethical committees as advised by the Medicines Commission are as follows (Baber, 1994):

• to require that trial applicants supply a certified statement that pre-clinical investigations have been carried out to a standard no less than that required by the Department of Health under the clinical trial exemption scheme (CTX); and in particular, because of the relevance to safety, that the quality and stability of the substance to be administered is assured

• 'to require, in submissions involving complex data, a succinct statement and/or an expert summary'

• 'to seek outside expert opinion if necessary'

- 'to refuse applications which make inadequate provision for compensation or injury due to participation'.

Other issues which need to be considered are gaining valid consent and the special needs of the mentally handicapped, Mental Health Act detainees, prinsoners, and minors under the age of 18.

The GP may also be approach by the researching unit for medical information on volunteers, e.g. for an opinion regarding the suitability of a patient to participate as a healthy volunteer. Important factors for the GP to consider are:

- past medical history of drug allergies
- asthma, hay fever or other evidence of atopy
- drug abuse, psychiatric history or alcoholism
- hospital consultations, surgical procedures or prosthesis
- hereditary and congenital malformations. For example, deafness associated with ECG QT prolongation abnormalities (Romano–Ward syndrome), although rare, may have important implications if undiagnosed, since the administration of an NCE which caused QT prolongation could precipitate a dangerous arrhythmia.

The importance of assessing volunteer suitability my be judged from the cynical definition of a healthy volunteer as 'a person who has been inadequately investigated', the presumption being that most people, if subjected to a detailed medical workup which includes 24 h ECG recording, full haematology and biochemistry profiles, together with a thorough clinical examination and history, would reveal some evidence of minor abnormality.

By volunteering for a drug trial, 'normal' people may therefore reveal hitherto unknown medical facts about themselves. For example, relatively common abnormalities discovered include ECG reports stating supraventricular tachycardia and accessory conduction pathways (e.g. Wolf–Parkinson–White syndrome) which may require further investigation and treatment.

Such unexpected findings require sensitive handling, with good communication between the clinical trial physician and the GP. Increasingly, CROs use local GPs recruited on a sessional basis to undertake medical examinations. This may, however, introduce potential conflict if clinical observations are revealed which affect life insurance risk or regulations associated with employment (an HGV licence, for example). The same strict rules regarding medical confidentiality apply and, in some cases, volunteers may decline to allow information to be passed to their employer or even their GP.

The GP as patient advocate

In the rare and unlikely event that a healthy volunteer is adversely affected by taking part in a trial, 'no fault' compensation should be available without admission of liability by the sponsoring pharmaceutical company or CRO. This cover also extends to the CRO, but will only apply if the incident occurred while the protocol was strictly followed and no negligence was involved. If negligent lack of care by the CRO is suspected, the GP may be approached by the patient to help in proving a case of medical negligence.

As with all cases of presumed medical negligence where mistakes may have been made, problems are often compounded by a lack of understanding and poor communication. As an independent party with responsibility for a patient's health and welfare, the GP may become an advocate for the patient.

Phase II studies

Phase II trials are principally designed to test for drug efficacy, provide data on safety and side effect (adverse event) profile, and produce an indication of drug dose ranges. The main objectives of phase II studies are to:

- reach a go/no-go efficacy decision
- define the minimum and maximum useful dose
- define likely clinical dose for pivotal efficacy studies
- estimate variability of clinical response to allow 'power and sizing' of phase III trials (i.e. have sufficient information to calculate the numbers of patients needed to test for statistical significance of the findings in the next phase of studies)
- form a basis for discussion with regulatory authorities.

Typically 100–300 patients will enter phase II trials. The phase II study population will be closely defined by the disease under investigation and will exclude high risk groups (such as the elderly and patients with cardiac, renal, and hepatic disease) from the protocol. Only after the safety profile and pharmacokinetics are defined in renal and hepatically impaired groups, and the metabolic fate of

Fig. 3.5 *Headache response to Zolmatriptan at hour 2*

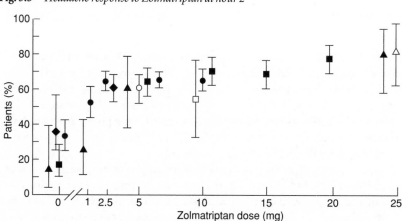

an NCE in humans is known with some certainty, will the protocol inclusion criteria be relaxed to include these groups.

If considered ethically acceptable, it is usual to carry out phase II trials using a parallel group design making comparisons with a randomized double blind placebo. Rescue medication (e.g. pain relief or other standard treatment) is usually permitted and may form one of the efficacy parameters. Figure 3.5 demonstrates a dose–response curve generated during phase II studies with Zolmatriptan, an orally active 5-HT agonist compound used to abort an acute migraine attack. Based on this data 2.5 and 5.0 mg were chosen as the clinically effective doses, with the best efficacy to adverse event ratio to proceed in pivotal phase III clinical trials.

During phase II the sponsoring company reaches a critical efficacy decision point (ED1) which is 'a point of no return'. The later a problem arises, the greater the investment lost if development is stopped. Withdrawal of a drug early, before phase II trials, based on a failure of concept, incurs relatively little

Fig. 3.6 *Compound attrition rates*

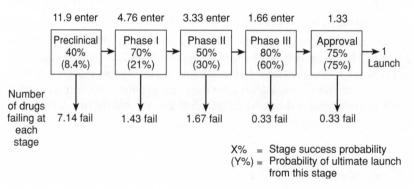

loss and is to be expected with 30% of NCEs (see Fig. 3.6). Withdrawal just before licensing may write off development costs in excess of £100 million.

The blocks of activity at the bottom of Fig. 3.2 emphasize the costly resource-intensive activities, such as long-term lifetime animal oncology studies and the other parallel activities (chemical plant manufacture and pharmaceutical development) which must be started immediately after ED1, if they are not to become become rate limiting factors for drug approval.

The commencement of phase II trials is a critical time for industrial regulatory interactions with the US Food and Drug Administration (FDA); with other national agencies, such as the UK Medicines Control Agency (MCA); and, more recently, with the newly formed European Medicines Evaluation Agency.

Fig. 3.7 *Discovery and development of a new medicine: regulatory interactions*

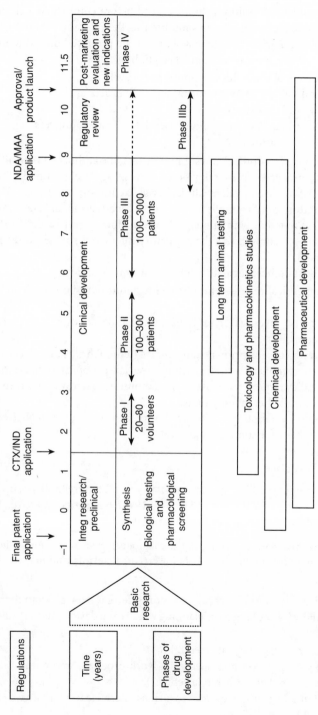

Plus: End of Phase II meetings
pre-NDA meetings
Manufacturing pre-approval inspection (PAI)...

Following the studies in healthy volunteers, and before commencing clinical studies in patients, a clinical plan is submitted to the relevant national drug agencies which summarizes the current status of the proposed drug development, together with supporting documents including:

- clinical trial protocol with ethics committee approval
- pharmaceutical stability, manufacturing and analytical data
- animal toxicity and exposure data
- summary of safety and likely maximum useful dose from volunteers
- statistical considerations.

Following review of the protocol and submitted data, the authorities then allow development to proceed. An Investigational New Drug Application (IND) is granted for the USA and equivalent Clinical Trial Exemption Certificate (CTX) for the UK. Statutory notification is then required for all serious adverse events within 3–10 days together with annual safety and efficacy review and further protocols. Figure 3.7 summarizes the regulatory interactions involved during drug development.

GP involvement in these regulatory interactions may be as:

- member of an ethical review committee with statutory responsibility under US law
- investigator or co-investigator responsible for study conduct and adverse event (AE) reporting
- principal investigator for primary care studies (although most practices will not be set up to run phase II studies without specialist support, because these early stage studies require particularly close monitoring and will often entail detailed blood and other investigations)
- holder of doctor's exemption certificate, if he or she is supplying an NCE on a named patient basis for compassionate use.

Good clinical practice

Good clinical practice (GCP) is an instrument to control the credibility of investigations for new drugs (Wallnofer and Cohen, 1993). Such attention to quality standards is enshrined in the European community GCP guidelines

... All parties involved in the evaluation of medical products share the responsibility of accepting and working according to Good Clinical Practice standards in mutual trust and confidence.

GCP compliance is now an integral part of any drug development programme and is essential to allow for the long term planning which drug development requires.
GCP provides for:

- rigid standardization giving data credibility
- standard operating procedures specifying work processes and clinical data collection (e.g. blood pressure measurement)
- independent quality assurance (QA), ensuring adherence to standards.

It is the duty of the pharmaceutical company to balance maintaining of the stable GCP environment (so that results obtained over the extended time frame of a drug development programme can be used for registration) against encouraging the scientific creativity of its investigators and employees to remain innovative in the long term.

Wallnover and Cohen (1993) use an excellent analogy to illustrate the importance employing trained clinical trial investigators, but at the same time formalize the process by the institution of GCP.

Imagine a pilot performing a routine landing with a commercial jet. During descent and landing he follows preset procedures providing the best conditions for a safe landing under normal conditions. This pilot now executes a highly formalized type of work which might be done by a much less skilled individual. Suddenly the four engines fail at the same time. The situation at once becomes highly dynamic and threatening. The pilot will still follow emergency procedures but he relies also on the integration and application of a lot of knowledge that is not covered by this procedure. For instance he knows he is flying in the proximity of a volcano and that volcanic ash may be the cause of his engine failure. He takes appropriate action and lands the plane safely. During this emergency his general professional training and experience has been more essential than formalized procedures.

GPs who become involved in clinical trials should make sure that they are aware of their obligations under GCP to:

- ensure that adequate time, facilities and staff are set aside if taking part in a study
- work with the company clinical research scientist to ensure data, information and documents are properly generated and recorded
- work according to SOPs and be prepared for QA inspection (external audit of the study)
- pay particular attention to drug accountability and patient identification.

Phase III: the pivotal clinical trials

Phase III trials usually involve 1000–3000 patients, at least some of whom will have received treatment for 1 year or more (i.e. at least 100 years' patient exposure). Most regulatory authorities require at least 'two well controlled confirmatory efficacy trials' which ideally should be placebo controlled. If this is not ethically acceptable, then comparison with the most widely registered clinical comparator is expected. This requirement can be problematic in international trials, where the same formulation of comparator is not available world-wide. The sponsoring company must then face reformulation of an existing product and matching placebo. This introduces the additional risk that the reformulated product may not be bioequivalent with respect to the marketed competitor.

The objectives of phase III trials are to:

- replicate and extrapolate efficacy in phase II trials using projected clinical dose
- demonstrate superiority or equivalence to placebo or active comparator

- provide confirmatory efficacy from two suitably powered clinical trials
- confirm the safety and tolerability profile in short term and long term use
- demonstrate a pharmacoeconomic benefit over established therapy.

In exceptional circumstances, and usually where there is evidence for a survival benefit or major distinguishing benefit of a new therapy over existing treatments, a single pivotal trial is considered acceptable. This is most likely to be observed for oncology drugs, for example bicalutamide (Casodex) 50 mg in combination therapy with castration in the treatment of carcinoma of the prostate was accepted by the FDA, and by other regulatory authorities worldwide, on the basis of one comparative study against flutamide with LHRH agonist (Fig. 3.8). In this study design Kaplan–Meier curve showed equivalent survival for the two treatments (Fig. 3.9), but bicalutamide was better tolerated (Fig. 3.10) with significantly fewer patients reporting diarrhoea ($p < 0.001$) (Schellhammer, 1996).

Fig. 3.8 *Trial randomization scheme for bicalutamide versus flutamide in prostatic cancer*

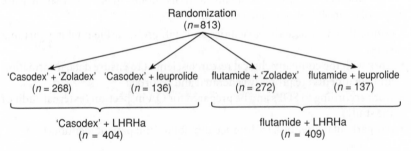

Following the satisfactory conclusion of Phase III trials, pre-NDA (new drug application) meetings are held with authorities. At this stage the authority will decide whether to fast track an application (6–9 months) if there is an important unmet medical need, such as drugs indicated for oncology or AIDS managements, or will elect to let the bureaucratic process take its course (18–24 months). In the US, where hearings are in public, patient pressure groups will often lobby the advisory boards for a speedy decision, with a resultant reduction in the review process.

The regulatory authorities will also conduct their pre-approval inspection (PAI) to ensure that the manufacturing facilities comply with internationally recognized good manufacturing practice (GMP). This not only means that the product meets tight analytical specifications but that the factory plants are 'environmentally friendly' and utilize the least hazardous manufacturing routes.

An important step for the company at this stage of drug development is to

Fig. 3.9 *The Kaplan–Meier probability of bicalutamide (-) versus flutamide (...) in prostatic cancer*

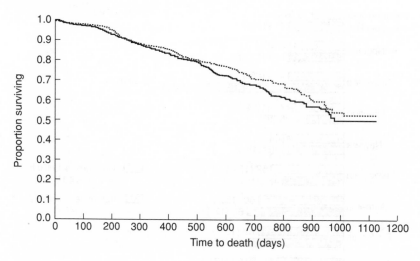

prepare high level documents which adequately represent safety (integrated summary of safety, ISS), efficacy (integrated summary of efficacy, ISE), together with an overall expert review of the product. The latter documentation is often produced by an independent expert. These documents are then filed with a pyramid of documents reflecting every pre-clinical and clinical report ever conducted with the compound. This may total over 200 volumes.

In addition to this paper mountain, all NDA dossiers are delivered as computer assisted NDAs (CANDAs) which allow authorities to interrogate the safety and efficacy databases, sometimes carrying out their own supplementary analyses. Thus the authorities can formulate their own views relative to the safety and efficacy data produced by the company.

Before review by the advisory boards, the company is given the opportunity to comment on the issues raised and to provide written or verbal replies to the agencies. In the USA the FDA meetings are usually open whereas currently in the UK the Committee on Safety of Medicines meets in closed session and reports to the MCA. The European Medicines Agency recently formed may play a role in arbitrating between different agency opinion in Europe via the CPMP. However, the system is still in its infancy and remains to be tried and tested.

Phase IIIb and Phase IV trials

Phase IIIb and Phase IV trials are designed to optimize the pre-marketing programme and to augment the brand as part of the life cycle management of a new treatment (see Fig. 3.11).

Fig. 3.10 *Adverse events reported in ≥10% of patients in either group that occurred during therapy (Zeneca Pharmaceuticals, data on file)*

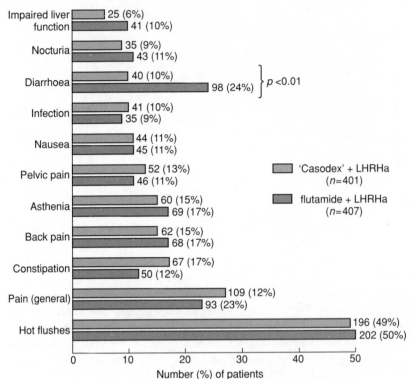

The medical department of an innovative company may deliver well-conducted trials, which appear to provide all the 'confidence' necessary for the rapid registration and adoption of medicines by the medical community. However, there continue to be significant delays in the adoption of new technology (including drugs) by doctors, for example, despite awareness of the importance of intravenous thrombolytics, uptake of new therapy had reached only 40% by 3 years after launch (Lancet editorial, 1993). Many of the factors involved in this gap between research evidence and implementation in practice are discussed elsewhere in this book. Therefore

although some well executed clinically relevant trials published in high profile journals have resulted in measurable changes in medical practice, others have exerted only limited influence, or none at all (Lancet Editorial, 1993).

With ABPI figures showing that only 1 in 4 NCEs provides a satisfactory return on investment, and with the growth phase of a product's life cycle being only 4.4 years, most commercial leverage needs to be applied early to guarantee

Fig. 3.11 *Customers buy augmented brands*

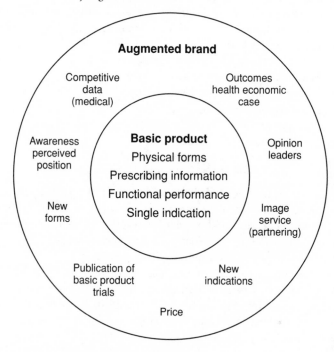

Basic product: Regulatory department
Augmented brand: Commercial development

Fig. 3.12 *New requirements for pharmaceutical marketing*

Traditional focus	Safety	Efficacy	Awareness	Cost effectiveness	Volume discount	Compliance	New needs
Physicians	X	X	X	X		X	
Regulators	X	X		X	X		
Pharmacists	X	X	X	X	X	X	
Managed care	X	X	X	X	X	X	
Pharm mgt co	X	X	X	X	X		
Patient	X	X	X			X	

New customers

recoupment of investment (Brown, 1994). The potential success of such marketing can be gauged by the pre-marketing of Serevent by Glaxo in the 1990s. An intensive educational and scientific programme resulted in almost 100% awareness of the product among GPs at launch, and an 80% 'ever usage' within 8 months. As in most areas of clinical practice, there are continual changes in emphasis required in marketing activities (Fig. 3.12).

Key factors which influence the design and conduct of IIIb and IV studies are:

- acceptance of concepts associated with new therapy
- relevance of innovation or advance to clinical usage
- favourable risk/benefit ratio for new product
- cost effectiveness and demonstrable healthcare benefit
- influence chain of opinion leaders acting as gate keepers.

Some IIIb trials may be carried out at the behest of regulatory agencies to address specific questions relating to efficacy or safety in special groups (e.g. studies in adolescents and children with innovative treatments for asthma and migraine). Post-marketing surveillance of certain class-related adverse events may be required to provide reassurance of long-term safety.

GPs may be approached to take part in phase IIIb or phase IV trials as part of the pre-marketing or post-launch marketing activity. The notorious 'seeding' studies should be a thing of the past, but GPs should ask themselves a number of questions before taking part in a phase IV study:

- will the study address valid clinical questions?
- does the study have unrestricted ethical approval?
- are the levels of funding commensurate with the work required (i.e. not excessive for the task and possibly an inducement to recruitment)?
- does it have Royal College approval?

Figure 3.13 illustrates a typical phase IV study which set out to evaluate once daily amlodipine in patients with isolated systolic hypertension, where the comparator drug was enalapril. Since both drugs were emerging as potential first line therapies, a direct comparison was considered to be clinically important because:

- different adverse event and efficacy profiles might suit different patient groups
- a study in primary care with home blood pressure recordings reflects 'real life' control.

A study such as this provides a good example of how a well-designed phase IV study can be carried out in a primary healthcare setting (Webster et al., 1993).

Summary

From a primary care perspective, drug development must deliver a cost-effective new therapy which meets an unmet medical need with either safety or efficacy advantages over existing treatments. As the main prescriber of any new medicine, the GP will need to assess the risk/benefit ratio relating to the new drug.

Fig. 3.13 *Mean (95% CI) changes from basline in supine systolic blood pressure recorded at clinic visit. Baseline (week 0) is the last weekly visit during the run-in phase on placebo. Week 10 represents the end of a 2 week washout period on placebo. Data relate to patients with complete results at each of the time points)*

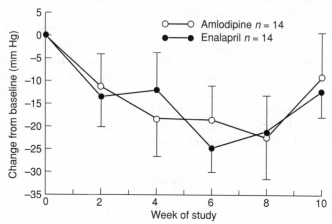

Fig. 3.14 *Average number of patients in clinical trials per NDA*

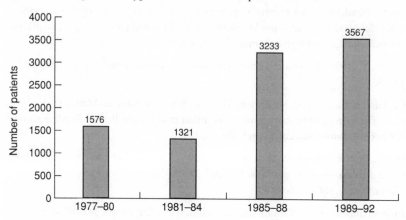

This applies not only in a medical context referring to side effects and toxicity, but is also about personal beliefs and concerns, which may relate to costs, peer pressure, and insecurity of trying a novel product before the decision to prescribe is made.

The pharmaceutical industry applies a different risk–benefit analysis covering two separate areas; company finance and patient welfare. The increasing numbers of patients needed to be exposed to novel compounds to satisfy regulatory bodies (Fig. 3.14), contributes to these costs and also the risks of developing drugs. Drug development is the largest financial undertaking for a research based company and can determine its success or failure. Withdrawal of a drug from the market and disappointing results with NCEs in its research portfolio can dramatically affect company share price.

For the primary care practitioner a knowledge of the drug development process provides an insight into the highly complex procedures needed to prepare the information relating to any product's potential risks and benefits as part of a licence application for a specified indication. At various stages during drug development the GP may also elect to become an investigator in clinical trials, or may become involved if one of their patients decides to volunteer. It is important to appreciate the differing objectives and involvement for each clinical phase, and to understand the implications for both patient and GP.

References

Arendt, J. (1995). Melatonin. *British Medical Journal,* **312,** 1242–3.

Baber, N. (1994). Volunteer studies: Are current regulations adequate? The ethical dilemma. *Pharmaceutical Medicine,* 8, 153–9.

Beaumont, G., Gringas, M., Hobbs, F. D. R., Drury, V. W. M. (1993). A randomised, double-blind, multi-centre, parallel-group study comparing the tolerability and efficacy of moclobemide and dothiepin hydrochloride in depressed patients in general practice. *International Clinical Psychopharmacology,* 7, 3/4, 159–65.

Brown, T. (1994). Constructing the right pre-marketing programme. *Scrip,* September, 12–15.

Gustafsson, C., Asplund, K., Britton, M., Norrving, B., Olsson, B., Marke, L.-A. (1992). Cost effectiveness of primary stroke prevention in atrial fibrillation: Swedish national perspective. *British Medical Journal,* **305,** 1457–8.

Hobbs, F. D. R., Aguado, A. G., Brumpt, I. (1996). Treatment of lower respiratory infections: a comparison of sparfloxacillin and clarithromycin. *First European Congress of Chemotherapy,* SECC, Glasgow.

Lancet Editorial (1993). Clinical trials and clinical practice. *Lancet,* 342(8876), 877–8.

Millson, D., Sohail, S., Lettis, S., Fenwick, S., (1992). Duration of inhibition of the flare response to intradermal 5-hydroxytryptamine in man by Alosetron (GR68755), a novel specific 5-HT3 receptor antagonist. *British Journal of Clinical Pharmacology,* **33,** 546P.

Minton, N. (1994). Volunteer models for predicting anti-emetic activity of 5-HT3-receptor antagonists. *British Journal of Clinical Pharmacology,* **37,** 525–30.

Orme, M., Harry, J., Routledge, P., Hobson, S. (1989). Healthy volunteer studies in Great Britain: the results of a survey into 12 months activity in this field. *British Journal of Clinical Pharmacology,* **27,** 125–33.

Schellhammer, P. (1996). Combined androgen blockade for the treatment of metastatic disease of the prostate. *Urology*, **47**, 622–8.

Wallnofer, A., Cohen, A. (1993). Good clinical practice: a question of balance. *British Journal of Clinical Pharmacology*, **35**, 449–50.

Webster, J. *et al.* (1993). A comparison of amlodipine with enalapril in the treatment of isolated systolic hyperetension. *British Journal of Clinical Pharmacology*, **35**, 499–505.

CHAPTER FOUR

Licensing and marketing of drugs

Michael Langman, Frank Wells, and Frank Leach

One inevitable consequence of drugs being developed by a commercial pharmaceutical industry is that, like other commodities, they are bought and sold for profit. However, they are a commodity with some very special features which make the market for drugs unique, in particular with regard to the extent to which it is stringently regulated. There are good reasons for the stringent regulation of the market in drugs. Firstly, drugs often require specialized information for their appropriate and effective use. Secondly, inappropriate use or misuse can have dangerous, even life threatening, consequences. Thirdly, the costs of drugs are often borne by parties other than the final consumers. In the case of the UK this is, by and large, the NHS, but in many other healthcare systems part or all of the costs of some or all of the drugs used by patients are paid for by third parties such as state or healthcare insurers.

Healthcare professionals, and especially doctors, have a special role in the drugs market because they possess the special knowledge required for the safe and effective use of drugs. This places responsibilities on doctors, in their role as proxy purchasers, to ensure that patients get the best medicine available for their condition and to select from the full range of possible products in a rational way. Doctors are also obliged, at the same time, to choose economically in order to protect their patients' interests as taxpayers. This, in effect, puts doctors in the position of rationers of health care either implicitly or, as is increasingly the case, explicitly. If doctors choose an unsafe or ineffective medicine they have failed in their duty of care towards their patients, and if they chose an unnecessarily expensive preparation for one patient other treatments may be denied other patients elsewhere—a concept known as 'opportunity costs' (see also Chapter 7).

The peculiar features of the drugs market also impose duties and obligations on other parties to the arrangement. Thus the pharmaceutical industry is expected to behave responsibly with regard to the marketing of its products. It is debarred, theoretically at least, from marketing directly to patients and can only market to doctors in their role as proxy consumers. Because of the special dangers of inappropriate use of drugs and the inability of individual consumers (either actual or proxy) to gauge the limitations of a product, pharmaceutical companies are expected to disclose fully any known hazards associated with the use of their products in addition to extolling their virtues. In the UK, the state is the major purchaser of pharmaceuticals and might be especially vulnerable to profiteering by the industry who, effectively, have a captive purchaser. The state, in the form of the Department of Health (DoH), has therefore negotiated a special arrangement with the industry to control the profits made from sales to the NHS. This arrangement, the Pharmaceutical Price Regulation Scheme, both limits and protects the profitability of the industry: this is particularly important in the UK, which has a large manufacturing pharmaceutical industry base making a substantial contribution to the overall economy.

The state, in its turn, also has responsibilities to ensure the best use of drugs. It has developed a particular role with regard to the safety of drugs use which is effected largely through a thorough and elaborate drug licensing process. This is most active at the point of introduction of the drug to the market place. The licensing system has to strike a careful balance between ensuring that dangerous or unhelpful drugs are not admitted to the market and yet ensuring that products that could benefit patients are not excluded unnecessarily or inadvertently. Once on the market, the drug's safety is monitored through various drug surveillance systems. The state also has a role in ensuring that doctors fulfill their responsibilities properly and are not improperly influenced by commercial or financial inducements and in ensuring the industry also behaves responsibly.

Drug licensing

Following the problems posed by the thalidomide disaster in the 1960s, the Medicines Act of 1968 was passed. This, in essence, set criteria of quality safety, and efficacy to be met if marketing approval were to be obtained in the UK. Applications for marketing licences are scrutinized by staff of the Medicines Control Agency, now a Crown Agency, which is responsible for ensuring that, apart from carrying out tasks related to medicines control, it can function within budgetary limits imposed by fee income collected during the licensing procedures.

Recent UK procedures

The procedures employed in licensing have, in essence, depended upon examination of dossiers provided by applicants. A view is then taken by agency staff. Where, for instance, new medicinal products are being considered, or where significant changes of use are being suggested, the provisional view of professional agency staff is taken through the advisory committee structure of the Agency, the Committee on Safety of Medicines (CSM). As a result the CSM has taken a definitive view which has usually been consonant with professional advice received. The definitive recommendations to Ministers vary from acceptance, to rejection, or provisional acceptance provided set conditions are met (for instance to restrict indications for use, or the dosage to be employed).

Companies have had the right to appeal and either to make written representations, or to present their case orally. The outcome can again vary from acceptance, to provisional acceptance, to rejection. Companies have then been able to appeal, if they so wished, to the Medicines Commission. Depending upon the outcome, a company may elect to be heard before a person appointed for the purpose by the licensing authority. The authority will then take account of that report in determining the outcome.

In essence, therefore, there are four possible stages resulting in advice to the licensing authority:

• initial CSM advice
• a hearing before the CSM
• appeal to the Medicines Commission
• a hearing before a person appointed for the purpose.

In this context it should be noted that the CSM is a committee composed of advisors chosen by reason of experience in the range of pharmacy, pharmacology, toxicology, clinical pharmacology, and therapeutics, and drawn generally from the staff of universities and the NHS. The Medicines Commission is more broadly based, including, for instance, industry representation, but with membership completely independent of the CSM. Persons appointed are again completely independent so that they can take a fresh view of whatever problem has arisen. In practice, most decisions are determined on the advice of the CSM alone, often after a hearing or written representations where issues have arisen.

When this licensing procedure was set up there was a clear need to consider the quality, safety, and efficacy of medicines already marketed, a task performed by the Committee on Review of Medicines. Outcomes were determined in much the same way as for newly marketed medicines.

Not all licensing matters have necessarily been put before expert committees for determination. Minor variations in drug formulation or in usage indications have been considered *ad hoc* by professional staff. The same has been true of applications for Clinical Trial Exemption certificates. It should be noted that these procedures apply to the licensing of prescription only medicines, and to more extended use, either through pharmacies or through general sale. The criteria employed will necessarily differ. Thus pharmacy and general sale imply self diagnosable conditions and the reasonable certainty of safe use without obtaining medical advice (see also Chapter 10).

Once licensing procedures have been satisfied and recommendations have been accepted there has remained a need to watch the outcome, in particular to determine if safety issues undetected at marketing authorization have arisen. In this context it has to be realized that only a few thousand individuals at most will have received a new medicine when marketing authorization is sought. Furthermore, although the potential for adverse effects, for instance in the very young or the very old, or in those taking other drugs, is explicitly considered during licensing, issues cannot all be foreseen. Adverse effects may, for instance, occur at a frequency of 1 in 1000 or less, thus being undetectable at marketing authorization. The complexities of ordinary clinical practice may also raise problems which could not be foreseen.

For such reasons a pharmacovigilance system was required so that safety problems could be detected as soon as possible. Furthermore, even if significant safety issues do not arise, the clinical position of a drug can change with time. Some become obsolescent and others develop differing indications. Licences have, therefore, been reviewed regularly on a 5-yearly basis.

The European dimension

The licensing of individual products separately in individual countries imposes an administrative and technical burden on agency staff in each country, but more especially on pharmaceutical companies seeking to market their products. The EU has therefore set up harmonization procedures, with a European Medicines Evaluation Agency, which is based in London and started operation in 1995. European procedures allow companies to seek licensing approval by two routes, one community-wide, and the other within individual countries.

The community procedures depend upon the nomination of a rapporteur state which is primarily responsible for the examination of the dossier produced by an individual company and the formulation of provisional recommendations. Other countries of the EU do, however, have the right to consider the same dossier and to form an independent view, usually formulated as reasoned objections. These responses are couched in terms allowing acceptance provided that objections which may be minor or major can be met. Thus major objections, if accepted, might effectively bar marketing authorization. The views of the rapporteur state and of the other member states are then brought together and a single synthetic view obtained, which, provided it is favourable, allows marketing authorization. Inevitably differences of opinion can arise, usually over minor issues, and satisfactory resolution has to be obtained. Nevertheless the system is only in its infancy and a definitive view is not yet obtainable.

The alternative procedure of licensing in a single state conforms in rough terms to the position prevailing under the UK Medicines Act of 1968 so that any definitive recommendation applies to the UK alone, but with European legislation overlying.

As in other spheres of EU legislation it is important to note that opting out is not possible. It is, therefore, important that the UK (and other states) clearly define issues of significance when new drug applications are made. The role of the Medicines Control Agency and of the expert committees associated remains undiminished, though altered in function.

Drug safety

Legislation and common sense dictate that drug safety is kept under review. In the UK the best known system has been that of spontaneous reporting of suspected adverse responses by doctors on 'yellow cards'. However, there are a variety of other methods. These include the examination of automated databases linking prescribing with outcome, periodic company safety updates, review of data obtained worldwide, and post-marketing surveillance.

The yellow card scheme

The yellow card system was set up over 30 years ago, and now generates some 20 000 reports each year, although it is important to realize that the method has strengths and weaknesses.

Firstly, reports are of suspected, not proven, adverse events (proof is necessarily difficult or impossible to obtain). As such they will consist of a mixture of true caused events and coincidental non-caused illnesses. Secondly, because reporting depends upon the perceptions of the reporter we cannot know what the true event rate is, though knowledge of total drug usage will allow a minimum rate for suspected (not necessarily caused) reactions to be estimated. Indeed, if every possible event was actively reported the scheme would collapse from overload. Past experience shows that reports are generated much less often for older than for newer drugs, that publicity given to potential problems generates more reports of the same, and that some doctors, notably those working in hospitals, are less likely to submit reports than GPs.

Differential reporting is actively encouraged by the 'black triangle' scheme. All new medicines have a black triangle placed beside their names in advertisements, in publications such as the BNF, and in their official descriptions. The triangle denotes a drug where all suspected adverse responses are to be reported, whether severe or trivial. This position contrasts with that for established drugs where the requirements are for reporting severe (even if well established) and previously unknown events.

The yellow card scheme has been very successful in identifying possible new risks, and emphasising the problems posed by those which have been established. Table 4.1 lists some of those successes in recent years. Data collected on yellow cards can be supplemented by world-wide reports, and is also made available by other routes, notably the WHO publication *Signal*. Occasionally these external reports denote risks not as yet detected in the UK, for instance those of cardiac arrhythmias in takers of cisapride or erythromycin together with the antifungals ketoconazole, itraconazole, and fluconazole.

Post-marketing surveillance

The systematic collection of data is another essential method of maintaining drug safety. Methods broadly depend upon the deliberate collection of cohorts of takers and examination of outcome. This can be done by deliberate special investigation, or by the use of automated databases. Whichever method is employed there is an associated requirement for comparator data so that observed rates or morbidity and mortality can be compared with expected population rates and/or with rates associated with the use of other drugs.

Table 4.1 *Adverse effects of drugs detected through UK spontaneous reports*

Drug	Adverse effects
Botulinum toxin	Dysphagia
Clozapine	Convulsions, myocarditis
Flecainide	Fibrosing alveolitis
High dose pancreatins	Ileocolonic strictures
Omeprazole	Diarrhoea
Paroxetine	Dystonia, withdrawal reactions
Remoxipride	Aplastic anaemia

In all such studies it is essential to remember that the format is not that of a randomized controlled trial. It cannot therefore be assumed that groups receiving and not receiving medicines under consideration are equivalent in all other respects. The conduct of such studies requires technical skill and commitment, and careful attention to design (Waller *et al.*, 1992). Guidelines on performing post-marketing surveillance have been published (Medicines Control Agency *et al.*, 1994).

Automated databases have been very valuable in identifying and confirming risks. Those available in the UK include the General Practice Research Database (formerly VAMP) and the Medicines Monitoring Unit in Dundee. The former has details on some 4 million patients registered with GPs throughout the UK, with outcomes (hospital referrals and admissions, deaths, chronic and recurrent diseases linked to drug use). The latter has details on practice prescriptions for some 400000 patients in Tayside and linked to hospitalization and deaths. The greater part of the information produced has been in response to possible safety issues—for instance the risks of gastrointestinal bleeding in takers of anti-inflammatory drugs, a hypothesis testing role which is that which one would expect. Comparison of data obtained in these databases with that obtained by other methods has shown generally consistent patterns.

Other data

Information obtained by spontaneous reporting and surveillance and special studies is supplemented by a variety of other information such as company's collections of data and time trend analyses—for instance, comparing the mortality from asthma (static) with the population use of ß-agonists (steeply rising) (Committee on Safety of Medicines 1992).

Methodological issues

In general terms there are three requirements in identifying safety issues.

- Is there a defined risk in terms of a rate per n (or n thousand) scripts issued?
- How much more frequent is that event than in non-users of the drug in question and/or in users of alternative medications for the same condition?
- Are there particular factors (such as age, concomitant disease and treatment) which materially influence risk?

Amongst the very large amounts of information available we can cite useful data on:

- the comparative risks of gastrointestinal bleeding in takers of anti-inflammatory drugs, with at least 10-fold variation
- the greater risk of dystonias in younger takers of metoclopramide
- the risks of mesalazine-associated blood dyscrasias—not very different from sulphasalazine in spontaneous reports, but quite different in database studies.

This illustrates the problems of spontaneous reports and possibly the restricted comparator in the database study (Bateman *et al.*, 1985; Langman *et al.*, 1994; Committee on Safety of Medicines, 1995).

Pharmacovigilance in Europe

The key principles of this European initiative are as follows. Firstly, member states will conduct pharmacovigilance studies and analyses within their own territories. However, those who hold marketing authorizations (generally pharmaceutical companies holding licences) are expected to operate pharmacovigilance systems and *inter alia* to report serious adverse drug reactions known to them within 15 days. Companies are also expected to provide safety updates at specified intervals and to respond to requests for safety information. Apart from these essentially passive roles they are expected to maintain risk–benefit evaluations and to take measures to improve produce safety.

The European Agency for the Evaluation of Medicinal Products (EMEA) has a co-ordinating role, and procedures exist to ensure that within the EU there is uniform action. This involves arbitration at the Committee on Proprietary Medicinal Products (CPMP). The procedure dictates that once a potentially serious safety problem has been detected in a particular country, other countries and EMEA should be told. This should occur before any material decision is taken. A rapporteur is then appointed to review the issues and report to CPMP. It should be emphasized, however, that in a case of urgency a member state can amend, suspend, or withdraw a licence summarily.

The procedures can be illustrated by events related to the possible risks of thrombo-embolism associated with the use of newer oral contraceptive agents reported in late 1995. (Jick *et al.*, 1995; WHO, 1995) On receiving information in the UK from several independent studies it was judged that a significantly enhanced risk of thrombo-embolism existed which was not balanced by attendant benefits. The CSM concluded that it was appropriate to restrict the recommended uses of the newer agents. The same information went to EMEA which, while accepting that there was evidence of risk, left it to member states to take such action they deemed necessary.

Marketing of drugs

From the above it is clear that the market in drugs is most tightly controlled at the point of entry to the market. However, other controls operate on the profitability of the industry supplying the market and on the promotion of drugs. These are now described.

The Pharmaceutical Price Regulation Scheme

The Pharmaceutical Price Regulation Scheme (PPRS) is an agreement between the UK Department of Health and the pharmaceutical industry, represented primarily by the Association of the British Pharmaceutical Industry (APBI). This scheme has the dual, seemingly disparate, purposes of securing safe and effective medicines for the NHS at reasonable prices while also promoting a strong pharmaceutical industry in the UK.

The formula under which the PPRS operates is complex, but it is based on tax returns and is a controlling mechanism which it is illegal to contravene. The PPRS sets a target profit for a pharmaceutical company, between 17 and 21% of the capital employed in the UK in providing those drugs. The target profit is not guaranteed: if a company exceeds the target by 25% or more, the Treasury may reclaim the excess profit, through taxation, while if a company underperforms by 25% (much rarer), the company will be permitted price rises. There is no regulation of individual drug prices in the PPRS, but only of overall profitability. What is not generally appreciated is that the scheme controls profits based on the whole portfolio of products marketed by the company to the NHS, not profits on individual items within that portfolio. Therefore a company may decide to price a handful of products at a level which hardly makes a profit at all so that other products can carry a higher profit margin. What matters is that the total amount of profit is within the permitted amount for that company during the year in question.

These controls contribute to assuring that expenditure in the UK on prescription medicines per person per year is much lower than in the USA or other major European countries including France, Italy, Germany, Belgium, and Spain, and is about the same as in the Netherlands. The negotiations with individual companies within this broad framework are confidential, and considerations include the contribution of the company to the UK economy as a whole, export earnings, and spending on research and development. The PPRS has been criticized particularly for this lack of transparency.

The PPRS is renegotiated regularly, not less than every 6 years, but more frequently if either the Government or the ABPI requests it 3 years after it was last renegotiated. In this context the ABPI represents the industry as a whole and it is appropriate at this stage to explain exactly what it does in all its various activities.

The Association of the British Pharmaceutical Industry

The ABPI represents 97% of the research-based pharmaceutical companies in the UK, and 85% of the generic companies. It looks after their interests *vis-à-vis* the Government and its various departments, including the DoH, the Treasury and the Department of Trade and Industry. The APBI represents not only UK parent companies—currently Glaxo-Wellcome, SmithKline Beecham, Zeneca and Fisons—but also virtually all the UK subsidiaries of multinational companies from the USA, Europe, and, now, Japan. It liaises closely with all interested parties, including most of the bodies representing the medical and pharmacy professions both collectively (e.g. the British Medical Association and the Royal Pharmaceutical Society of Great Britain) and by specialty (e.g. the medical Royal Colleges, Association of Professors of Clinical Pharmacology).

The Association was formed in 1930 and was responsible in 1958 for drafting a Code of Practice for the Pharmaceutical Industry. This code, drawn up and constantly revised in consultation with the British Medical Association, the Royal Pharmaceutical Society of Great Britain and the Medicines Control Agency (previously the Medicines Division) of the DoH, effectively acts as the set of rules under which pharmaceutical companies conduct their promotional activities. It is a condition of membership of the ABPI to abide by the code in both the spirit and the letter. Companies which are not members of the Association may give their formal agreement to abide by the code and accept the jurisdiction of the independent Prescription Medicines Code of Practice Authority. Over 50 companies have done so, and the code is therefore accepted by virtually all pharmaceutical companies operating in the UK. It is important that doctors, pharmacists, and the British public are aware that the code exists, is used, and is internationally generally reckoned to be rigorous.

The APBI produces guidelines and information documents on a large number of topics relevant to the pharmaceutical industry such as on good clinical research practice, clinical trial compensation, clinical trial audit, drafting of patient information leaflets, conduct of market research and so on. The association also publishes two compendia which are sent to all GPs, hospitals, hospital pharmacies and community pharmacies; the Compendium of Data Sheets and Summaries of Product Characteristics, and the Compendium of Patient Information Leaflets (Association of the British Pharmaceutical Industry, 1995a, 1995b).

The Compendium of Data Sheets and Summaries of Product Characteristics, though bulky, is the only volume which brings together data sheets and summaries of product characteristics for virtually all medicinal products. Data sheets and summaries of product characteristics are the statutory documents providing information to prescribers which has to be in line with the conditions of the product licence for each medicinal substance given marketing authorization.

The role of advertising

There is a role for the advertising of medicines as, without promotion, none of us would be other than marginally aware of what was available in any field. Any commodities, be they cars, food products, cosmetics, or computers need to be promoted. Promotional activites by the pharmaceutical industry are directed mainly at information about new products, or new indications for existing drugs, and what is currently available. Doctors and pharmacists need to make critical analyses of what they are told, from whatever source, and the promotional activities of pharmaceutical companies readily fall into the Code of Practice for the Pharmaceutical Industry analytical process.

One of the objectives of the Code of Practice for the Pharmaceutical Industry is to ensure that the promotion of medicines to members of the health professions and to appropriate administrative staff is carried out in a responsible, ethical and professional manner, so that the critical analysis referred to above can be much more easily achieved than would apply if the code did not exist. The code therefore recognizes and seeks to achieve a balance between the needs of patients, doctors, pharmacists, and other health professionals, the general public and the industry regarding the need to disseminate information within the political and social environment in which the industry operates and the statutory controls which exist governing the marketing of medicines. What this means is that the industry has to do its level best to abide by the rules, otherwise it will be penalized. The existence of the Code of Practice does not, of course, relieve doctors of their individual ethical and legal responsibilities to resist inappropriate marketing and to prescribe responsibly in the best interest of patients uninfluenced by commercial pressure or the prospect of personal gain.

The prescriber's response to drug advertising

Doctors (and other health professionals) are exposed to the promotional activities of the drug industry in many and diverse ways. Such activities are familiar and commonplace. Medical journals and newspapers (especially those which depend heavily on advertising revenue) invariably contain colourful and seductive drug advertisements, many of which portray impressive marketing skills. Similar 'glossies' pass, in unending succession, through the family doctor's letter box. The visit of the drug representative (often armed with voluminous brochures), the lunchtime presentation, audiovisual packages, and even exotically sited symposia all provide useful alternatives routes to the 'brain-store' of the prescriber.

Doctors may argue that they are immune to such ploys, but the large amount of money devoted by a highly successful industry to drug promotion suggests that it yields financial rewards. The distribution of gifts to doctors is now stringently controlled by the ABPI Code of Practice, and those gifts that do escape censure are often clearly marked with the brand name of a product, thus providing a subtle but effective *aide-memoire*.

Promotion of drugs via the patient is an alternative approach which may easily avoid official scrutiny. Doctors and health issues are popular subjects for the media and articles on the latest 'wonder cure' may lead to the exertion of patient pressure on a GP for a prescription. Similarly, successful promotion of a new drug to hospital consultants, especially when at substantial discount, can lead to referred prescribing by GPs. The latter factor may increase in importance with the reduced influence of drug and therapeutics committees in response to the internal market and the devolution of budgetary responsibilities to individual clinical entities.

The popular view that promotional excesses of the drug industry are countered by the altruism, authority, and independence of the medical journals is comfortable but often inaccurate. Concern has been expressed, for example, that seemingly independent medical reviews, even when published in eminent journals, can be covert forms of drug promotion (Smith, 1994) while the poor quality of many published drug trials (see below) can raise suspicions concerning the motives underlying their publication. Articles in journal supplements may be particularly deserving of careful evaluation since these may lack even the minimal safeguard of peer review (Rochon *et al.*, 1994).

Psychological factors in drug advertising have been the subject of recently published investigations by Kincey *et al.* (1994). Seemingly irrelevant details in an advertisement, such as differences in text size, can greatly influence the perception of a message by the casual observer and it is noteworthy that concern at the illegibility of 'sensitive' sections of drug advertisements (i.e. those dealing with prescribing details) has been expressed (Collier and New, 1984). The maxim that a picture can convey more than words is thoroughly exploited by advertisers. For example, the glamorous, successful, and attractive young women portrayed in advertisements for the contraceptive pill contrast sharply with the appearance of the harassed mother of a large family who has escaped the protective influence of exogenous hormones. An additional observation is that subjects depicted in drug advertisements are usually clean, attractive, and conventional in appearance. They are people to whom members of a correspondingly conventional and middle-class profession can easily relate.

A cardinal first move in assessing claims made for an individual drug is to attempt to 'define the message'. The prescriber might ask if a distinct claim is being made in terms of safety, efficacy, or other relevant factors, or whether the promotion is merely a bland reminder of a drug's existence. Particular care should be exercised in response to claims for therapeutic 'selectivity' (rarely if ever absolute) or 'potency', which usually has more relevance to the laboratory than to clinical practice. The evidence for the value of sustained-release preparations should be based on realistic comparisons with standard formulations of the same drug and should relate to the clinical response of patients rather than solely to pharmacokinetic data. Non-sequiturs are by no means uncommon and typically include the unjustified extrapolation of laboratory data to clinical practice.

When drug advertisements do include references, these may be liberally sprinkled with citations of 'data on file', 'to be published', or 'symposium proceedings'. Although they are not necessarily flawed, such sources should not be accepted without inspection. If original papers are available, it is useful to compare the authors' conclusions with the claims made in the relevant advertisement. English is a language which is particularly amenable to subtle manipulation and instances are not unknown of discrepancy between the claims in an advertisement and the contents of references which it cites.

Wade *et al.* (1989), in an Australian study, approached 10 international companies with a request to supply their best evidence in support of marketing claims for 17 products. The authors concluded from their investigation that the standards of evidence used to justify advertising claims are inadequate. In a similar vein, Herxheimer *et al.* (1993) surveyed advertisements for medicines in leading medical journals in 18 countries over 12 months. They noted that generic names usually appeared in smaller type than did brand names. Indications were mentioned more frequently than negative effects, important warnings and precautions were missing in half the samples and contraindications in about 40%. It was suggested that

if advertisements are not considered seriously they will influence the use of medicines, as they are intended to do, but that read critically they can provide useful information.

A detailed discussion on the evaluation of clinical trials would be outside the context of this chapter and excellent summary guidelines have, in any case, been published elsewhere (Anon, 1985a,b). The correspondence columns of medical journals are frequently occupied by controversies relating to this important theme. Defects in trial design, analysis, and interpretation are not infrequent and are a justifiable cause for concern. Even the comparatively novel and powerful tool of meta-analysis can yield results which conflict with those of subsequent mega-trials (Anon, 1995). Since the promotion of drugs commonly rests on the authority of published papers it is wise to be circumspect about the uncritical acceptance of such evidence without adequate evaluation or access to peer review. The results of trials using placebo controls, while of value in the early stages of a drugs evaluation, are generally less informative than those with pharmacologically active controls.

The graph (as well as the histogram, pie-chart, and bar-chart) can provide a colourful and concise summary of data in drug advertisements but needs careful assessment since its defects may only become apparent after some reflection. The discerning observer may note the absence of labelling of axes or failure of such axes to start at zero (leading potentially to axial distortion). These anomalies and the use of 'amputated' bar charts (i.e. those which do not extend to zero) can yield misleading comparisons. 'Assumption of linearity', by drawing a straight line through two solitary points on a graph, may convey an erroneous impression of a neat and consistent relationship between two variables. Use of error bars to qualify plots of mean values needs critical assessment but when used correctly can usefully indicate the precision of the relevant data.

The statistical content of drug advertisements is usually confined to quotation of probability (p) values. The smaller the p value the less chance there is that the observed results have arisen by chance. That, at least, is the theory. The objective of using inferential statistical tests is to ascribe to a set of results an estimate of reliability. To be valid, such testing demands application of an appropriate test to correspondingly appropriate data. This empirical precaution may commonly be disregarded. Furthermore, statistical significance does not necessarily denote clinical significance. Even simple summary statistics such as the average (mean) may be seriously disturbed by one or two atypical outliers, hence the value of confidence intervals. The use of percentages to disguise small sample sizes is equally reprehensible. It is also useful to be on the lookout for conversion of crude descriptive measures of response (e.g. slight, moderate, severe) into numerical values (i.e. 1, 2, 3) which can yield results with a false impression of precision.

A review by Herxheimer and Collier (1990) of complaints regarding drug advertising made to the ABPI Code of Practice Committee between 1983 and 1988, revealed that the majority came from doctors and competing companies. Their overall conclusion that 'the rules that forbid misleading or unsubstantiated information and misleading claims or comparisons are broken most often' is a salutary reminder of the need for vigilance. Their view, that the Code of Practice Committee should become publicly accountable, that the majority of its members should represent the public and the professions and that effective sanctions are needed provides a fruitful basis for debate.

Relationships between doctors and the pharmaceutical industry

The promotional effects of the pharmaceutical industry, of course, go beyond just advertising their products. Other aspects of the relationships between the industry and the healthcare professions are also governed by the Code of Practice for the Pharmaceutical Industry. Thus there are stipulations regarding the conduct and training of company representatives, the provision to professionals of samples and gifts, the provision of hospitality and the hosting or sponsoring of meetings. All healthcare professionals should be aware of what is and is not allowed under the Code of Practice. Healthcare professionals are also offered guidance on how to conduct their relationships with industry (BMA, 1993; GMC, 1996). These guidelines correspond closely to the Code of Practice, so they are mutually reinforcing. For instance, the Code of Practice states that members of health professions will not be offered gifts or inducements to prescribe particular products, while the General Medical Council guidance to doctors advises against accepting gifts or inducements. Both codes of behaviour allow the giving and receiving of gifts of nominal value relevant to the doctor's work. The industry and the professions enjoy considerable trust vested in them by the general public, who are naturally perturbed when breaches of these self-imposed codes of conduct occur. It is important to the continuation of this bond of trust that both parties see to it that their respective codes of conduct are adhered to. Representatives of the industry should be prepared to report improper behaviour by health professionals to their governing bodies, and likewise health professionals are duty bound to report breaches of the Code of Practice to the ABPI.

References

Anon (1985a). Reading between the lines of clinical trials—1: design. *Drug and Therapeutics Bulletin*, **23**, 1–3.

Anon (1985b). Reading between the lines of clinical trials—2: analysis. *Drug and Therapeutics Bulletin*, **23**, 5–7.

Anon (1995). Magnesium, myocardial infarction, meta-analysis and megatrials. *Drug and Therapeutics Bulletin*, **33**, 25–7.

Association of the British Pharmaceutical Industry (1995*a*). *Compendium of Data Sheets and Summaries of Product Characteristics*. Datapharm Publications, London.

Association of the British Pharmaceutical Industry (1995*b*). *Compendium of Patient Information Leaflets*. Datapharm Publications, London.

Bateman, D. N., Rawlins, M. D., Simpson, J. M. (1985). Extrapyramidal reactions with metoclopramide. *British Medical Journal*, **291**, 930–2.

BMA (1993). *Medical ethics today: its practice and philosophy*, pp. 295–8. BMJ Publishing, London.

Collier, J., New, L. (1984). Illegibility of drug advertisements. *Lancet*, **1**, 341–2.

Committee on Safety of Medicines and Medicines Control Agency (1995). Blood dyscrasias and mesalazine. *Current Problems in Pharmacovigilance*, **21**, 5–6.

Committee on Safety of Medicines (1992). Beta-agonist use in asthma: report from the CSM Working Party. *Current Problems*, **33**, 1–2.

GMC (1996). *Good medical practice*. General Medical Council, London.

Herxheimer, A., Lundborg, C. S., Westerholm, B. (1993). Advertisements for medicines in leading medical journals in 18 countries: a 12-month survey of information content and standards. *International Journal of Health Services*, **23**, 161–71.

Herxheimer, A., Collier, J. (1990). Promotion by the British Pharmaceutical Industry, 1983–8; a critical analysis of self regulation. *British Medical Journal*, **300**, 307–11.

Jick, H., Jick, S. S., Gurevich, V., Wald Myers, M., Vasilakic, C. (1995). Risk of idiopathic cardiovascular death and non-fatal venous thrombo-embolism in women using oral contraceptives with differing progestagen components. *Lancet*, **346**, 1589–93.

Kincey, J., Saltmore, S., Leach, F., Bradley, C. (1994). Content and persuasion strategies in drug information leaflets sent to general practitioners: a pilot analysis. *Health Psychology Update*, **18**, 6–9.

Langman, M. J. S., Weil, J., Wainwright, P., Lawson, D. H., Rawlins, M. D., Logan, R. F. A., Murphy, M., Vessey, M. P., Colin Jones, D. G. (1994). Risks of bleeding peptic ulcer associated with individual non-steroidal anti-inflammatory drugs. *Lancet*, **343**, 1075–8.

Medicines Control Agency, Committee on Safety of Medicines, Royal College of General Practitioners, British Medical Association, and Association of the British Pharmaceutical Industry (1994). Guidelines for company-sponsored safety assessment of marketed medicines (SAMM guidelines) *British Journal of Clinical Pharmacology*, **38**, 95–7.

Rochon, P. A., Gurwitz, J. H., Cheung, M., Hayes, J., Chalmers, T. (1994). Evaluating the quality of articles published in journal supplements compared to the quality of those published in the parent journal. *Journal of the Americal Medical Association*, **272**, 108–13.

Smith, R. (1994). Conflict of interest and the *British Medical Journal*. *British Medical Journal*, **308**, 4–5.

The Medicines for Human Use (Marketing Authorisations Etc) Regulations (1994). Statutory Instruments No. 3144.

Wade, V. A., Mansfield, P. R., McDonald, P. J. (1989). Drug companies evidence to justify advertising. *Lancet*, **2**, 1261–3.

Waller, P. C., Wood, S. M., Langman, M. J. S., Breckenridge, A. M., Rawlins, M. D. (1992). Review of company post-marketing surveillance studies. *British Medical Journal*, **304**, 1470–2.

World Health Organization (1995). Collaborative Study of Cardiovascular Disease and Steroid Hormone Contraception. I: venous thrombo-embolic disease and combined oral contraceptives; results of international multicentre case-control study *Lancet*, **346**, 1575–82.

CHAPTER FIVE

How doctors choose drugs

Petra Denig and Colin Bradley

Prescribing drugs is a routine behaviour for most doctors. Many prescriptions are written during consultations, apparently without the doctor giving it much thought. However, each time a prescription is written a decision has been made. This decision making can be considered from a prescriptive or normative point of view; discussing how doctors ought to choose drugs and the factors that properly ought to influence that process. Such an approach would deal with questions of diagnostic decision making and statements regarding the optimal drug treatment for problems presenting in primary care. These questions, though, are beyond the scope of this book and are properly addressed in textbooks of medicine and therapeutics. This chapter is concerned rather with the descriptive domain of decision making and seeks to describe how the decisions are actually made by doctors, rather than how they ought to be made.

The reasons for offering this description of prescribing decisions are twofold. Firstly, recent research has improved our understanding of these processes. Secondly, if we have a better understanding of how decisions are actually made, we can advise more authoritatively on how prescribing decisions can be improved. However, before considering how drugs are chosen once the decision to prescribe has been made, we shall consider the issues around the decision to prescribe in the first place.

Pressures on prescribing

The first choice a doctor makes when considering possible therapeutic responses to a patient's problem is the decision of whether a drug is required at all (Bradley, 1991). This decision is particularly a feature of therapeutic decision making in the primary care setting where the possibility of not prescribing a drug is much more likely to constitute the clinically appropriate response. This is because problems presenting in primary care are more likely to represent manifestations of 'non-illness' (i.e. symptoms in the absence of demonstrable disease).

Furthermore, for many of the self-limiting diseases presenting in primary care there is no specific therapy that will alter the course of the disease and the best that can be offered is some non-specific remedy to reduce symptoms. Finally, even where the patient has significant disease for which there is specific therapy, the probability is greater in primary care that the disease will be at the milder end of the disease spectrum, where the balance of safety and efficacy of drug treatment might still favour no treatment. Thus, for instance, elderly women presenting in general practice with 'arthritis' in whom a non-steroidal anti-inflammatory drug (NSAID) would undoubtedly give some relief of symptoms might not be prescribed one because the substantial risk of gastro-intestinal side effects outweighing any benefit.

One might, therefore, expect that consultations in primary care would commonly end without any prescription being issued. Figures for the proportion of consultations ending without a prescription do not, however, entirely bear out this presumption. Furthermore, GPs describe themselves as being under considerable pressure to prescribe, even when this is against their better judgment. In a study of prescribing decisions with which the doctor admitted some discomfort (Bradley, 1992), doctors describe feeling pressurized into prescribing by a variety of other influences, including the expectations of the patient, precedents set by colleagues prescribing, and concerns about the possible effect of not prescribing on the doctor–patient relationship. These pressures to prescribe can, therefore, be identified as coming from three main sources: patients, doctors, and the pharmaceutical industry. More recently, a countermanding pressure to avoid prescribing wherever possible has come from those responsible for the funding of healthcare, i.e. governments and health insurers.

In addition to these external pressures to prescribe, doctors place internal pressures on themselves; for instance, time pressure to end the consultation may lead to a prescription. Pressure to avoid difficult or uncomfortable dealings with a patient may also lead to a prescription rather than a fraught consultation (Balint et al., 1970). The doctor's need to fulfil his or her role has also been perceived as leading to a prescription, as it is difficult to justify one's status as a healer if one offers no concrete manifestation of treatment (Hall, 1980).

Pressure from patients

Several studies have shown how doctors clearly perceive a great demand from patients for medication. However, research indicates that the doctors may overestimate this patient demand (Bradley, 1992; Britten, 1994). Several studies have identified a mismatch between the frequency with which doctors anticipate a patient demand for medication and the frequency with which patients will admit to having such a desire. Indeed, Virji and Britten (1991) have shown how a proportion of patients are actually 'drug averse', a possibility not usually even entertained by their doctors.

When asked how they know patients are expecting a prescription, doctors refer to a variety of behaviours by their patients which they interpret as signalling a desire for a medication (Bradley, 1990). Doctors have described overt requests for a prescription from patients such as the direct question 'Aren't you going to give me something, then?' But other more subtle patient behaviours are also interpreted as constituting pressure to prescribe. The patient looking crestfallen during the consultation can be taken to indicate an unexpressed desire for medication; so can a patient choosing to see a different doctor in the practice; or calling out a doctor out of hours; or threatening the doctor with reporting to the authorities or even physical violence; or repetition of the presenting complaint after no prescription is offered; and so on.

While all these may be signals of dissatisfaction, there is often a presumption on the part of doctors that the dissatisfaction is related to whether or not medication was prescribed, which may not be the case at issue. The characteristics of the patients who are alleged to pressurize the doctor to prescribe have also been identified. Doctors report having more difficulty refusing prescriptions to patients who are very young or very old, patients who belong to ethnic minorities, patients whom they know very well or not at all (such as temporary residents), and patients for whom they have a strong affinity or a strong disdain. It has also been shown how this perceived overprescribing is related to the nature of the drug under study and the disease, and a number of other less easily explained factors such as whether or not the patient had an appointment (Virji and Britten, 1991).

Pressure from other doctors

In a study of uncomfortable prescribing decisions, the effect of precedent was identified as one of the major sources of pressure to prescribe when the doctor did not really want to (Bradley, 1992). It appears that precedents, once set, are very difficult to alter. Precedents could be set by a hospital doctor, by another doctor working in the practice, or sometimes even by the prescribing doctor him- or herself in a previous encounter with the patient. There appear to be particularly difficulties to be overcome in trying to break with each of these three sources of precedent. In relation to hospital colleagues, difficulties arise from the immense faith patients often have in the word of the specialist. For a GP to go against specialist advice seems, to the patient, at best, pointless (i.e. why refer if you are not going to take the advice offered) and, at worst, positively foolhardy.

Precedents set by practice colleagues are difficult to break because of the readiness with which one's colleagues are able to observe your prescribing and comment on it. Differences between doctors in their prescribing for the same condition are highlighted and can, potentially at least, lead to conflict between doctors as well as a loss of face in front of the patient. Finally, there are difficulties in seeking to break a precedent set by yourself because of concerns that to vary prescribing policy from one occasion to the next would seem to the patient rather inconsistent and indecisive.

Pressure from the pharmaceutical industry

The pharmaceutical industry invests large sums in marketing, particularly to doctors (see Chapter 4). The companies would argue that they market only particular products and then only for their licensed indications. However, the intensity of drugs marketing is such that it is likely to have a more general effect on promoting the idea of there being a medicine for every ailment and, hence, promoting the use of drugs in general. There is an obvious parallel here with the marketing of cigarettes and tobacco products, which manufacturers argue is solely about dividing up market share but, in reality, has been shown to relate also to the general level of consumption.

Drug companies also support campaigns that bring certain diseases or issues to the attention of the prescribers (and patients), thus encouraging the treatment of those diseases. For example, a programme that stimulates cholesterol screening encourages a perceived need for lipid lowering drugs. There are also anecdotal reports of doctors being more directly pressurized to prescribe drugs and the concerns over some post-marketing surveillance studies, so called 'seeding trials', being little more than thinly veiled marketing ploys.

Pressures to not prescribe

A relatively new development in the prescribing field has been the increasing involvement of healthcare funders in seeking to influence prescribers, usually in the direction of moving away from prescribing drugs. Just as there are risks in prescribers being pressurized into prescribing when this is not clinically appropriate, there are also risks in being pressurized into not prescribing when it is appropriate to prescribe.

Prescribers need to be clear about why they chose to prescribe in each case and what the net benefits accruing to patients are intended to be. There is an increasing pressure on all professions to be more accountable. Thus doctors need to be able to account for the expenditure incurred as a result of their prescribing and this needs to be justified on the grounds of being a better use of the resources available than any alternative use to which those resources might be put. Making this case, which is essentially establishing the cost-effectiveness of treatment, requires some expertise in health economics. One of the implications of the current climate of financial stringency and increased professional accountability is that doctors will need to learn the skills necessary to mount an economic as well as a clinical defence of their prescribing decisions (see Chapter 7).

Choosing between different drugs

Most doctors would like to believe that once they have decided to prescribe, choosing a drug treatment for a patient is the result of a controlled and reasoned decision process in which the best option is selected following a comparison and evaluation of all possible treatment options on their benefits and costs. In practice, doctors may follow a number of alternative decision strategies. Which strategy is followed varies as a function of the task, the context and the decision maker. Some situations elicit a very deliberate balancing of pros and cons, whereas in other cases simple decision rules are being followed. As well as the situation determining which decision strategy is followed, the use of a particular strategy can also be in part a characteristic of a particular doctor. Before describing the possible decision strategies we will first consider the formal decision analytic approach.

Decision analysis

There is a systematic, explicit, and quantitative approach to decision making which is known as decision analysis. Although there is controversy over the utility and feasibility of using decision analysis in medical practice, this approach is becoming more common for making, for instance, formulary decisions (Summers & Szeinbach, 1993).

Table 5.1   *Five steps in decision analysis*

Step 1	Define the problem and the objectives
Step 2	Structure the decision problem; identify all possible alternatives and relevant decision criteria
Step 3	Estimate the probability that a particular option will lead to a specific outcome
Step 4	Evaluate the attractiveness or value of each possible outcome
Step 5	Choose the best option by combining probabilities and values

In Table 5.1 the different steps of a decision analysis are presented (Abelson & Levi, 1985). After identification of the problem and the objectives (step 1), one has to structure the decision problem. Which alternative options should be considered, and what are the relevant decision criteria (step 2)? From a theoretical point of view, outcomes such as efficacy, side effects and cost are seen as relevant criteria for treatment decisions. Then information is needed to fill in the structure (step 3).

For each possible option, estimates must be made of its outcomes. Furthermore, the attractiveness or value of each of those outcomes must be determined (step 4). In other words, how important is it to have an effective treatment or a safe treatment or a cheap treatment? Then the risks and benefits can be balanced, and the treatment with the highest overall value selected (step 5). Thus the final decision is made in a so-called maximizing strategy. It is important to realize that in this type of decision strategy all treatment outcomes are weighed simultaneously and therefore positive outcomes can compensate for negative ones.

83

Personal set of drugs

Decisions made in practice do not follow a clear stepwise and quantitative approach such as that described above. First of all, doctors seldom consider all possible alternatives. It is not feasible for a GP to know all details of all treatments available on the market. Therefore, each doctor has a personal set of drugs with which he or she is familiar and normally chooses from when confronted with an individual patient. The personal selection (set) of a GP will typically include 150–200 different drugs (Taylor and Bond, 1991). When confronted with a specific patient case, only a few drugs will come into mind, i.e. the so-called 'evoked set'. Depending on the diagnosis, the average number of drugs in the evoked set varies between two and five (Denig, 1994).

Therefore, the doctor makes two types of decision. The first is the decision whether to adopt a (new) drug to this personal set. The second is the decision to choose a particular drug from this set for an individual patient. For both decisions a number of different decision strategies can be followed. Some strategies can be seen as variations on the decision analytic approach, i.e. trading off the benefits and risks of different treatments in a maximizing strategy.

Other strategies that have been identified in medical practice are essentially different from the decision analytic approach. Driven by pragmatism, intuition, or emotions, doctors may use simple decision rules and shortcuts that make the decision process easier and faster. All these variations and shortcuts do not necessarily lead to inappropriate drug choices, but they do explain why there is so much variation in prescribing decisions in practice. These various strategies are now discussed in more detail.

Decision strategies in practice

The analytic approach

When questioned, doctors usually say that their treatment decisions are based on a trade-off involving a number of medical and pharmaceutical outcomes. They have certain expectations about the drug treatments, and—at least implicitly—assign different values to each of the treatment outcomes. Doctors report that they try to find the best treatment for a patient using these expectations and values. Such a decision strategy could be seen as a variation on the decision analytic approach, and is therefore called the 'analytic approach'. Although this may partly reflect a tendency to give a professionally desirable explanation, it seems that this kind of decision making does actually occur in practice.

Using this concept of expectations and values, a model has been developed by researchers to describe and predict the treatment choices of doctors (see Box 5.1) (Denig & Haaijer-Ruskamp, 1992). This model can be expected to predict drug choices correctly in 3 out of 4 cases if the doctor's personal expectations and values are included. One must keep in mind that those expectations and values are not necessarily adequate from a theoretical point of view. The model assumes that the doctor tries to make a balanced decision, but may of course make errors in his or her judgments or evaluations.

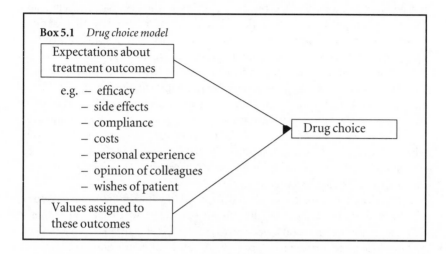

Box 5.1 *Drug choice model*

Expectations about treatment outcomes

e.g. – efficacy
     – side effects
     – compliance
     – costs
     – personal experience
     – opinion of colleagues
     – wishes of patient

Values assigned to these outcomes

Drug choice

To make an analytically reasoned decision the doctor first has to determine which criteria (which treatment outcomes) are relevant for his or her decision. There are many possible decision criteria. Doctors perceive the following to be relevant pharmacological and economic criteria:
• efficacy
• side effects
• compliance (e.g. convenience of dosage schedule and administration)
• cost
Other less cognitive aspects reported to be of influence are:
• patient's wishes
• perceived professional acceptability
• personal experience.

Doctors seldom use all the criteria that they claim as being relevant for all decisions. In general, it has been found that most decision makers effectively use only four or five criteria for their decision. Once they have decided which aspects are relevant for the decision, they must make estimates of how the different options would score on these aspects. Often only rough estimates are made by doctors, such as this drug is 'quite effective' or 'extremely effective' or 'more effective in comparison to another drug'. In other words, they seldom quantify the exact probabilities of a treatment outcome.

When doctors do quantify those probabilities, their estimates are often not in accordance with the available (scientific) knowledge. There is a large variation in what doctors expect of specific treatments. While some believe a particular drug is effective for only 40% of a certain group of patients, others believe that 90% of these patients would benefit from the treatment (Denig, 1994). Also, large differences in expectations are encountered with regard to side effects and costs.

This variation is the result of a number of biases. The information doctors receive may be incomplete or biased. In addition, the doctors themselves are selective when collecting information; sometimes information is collected only to seek confirmation of pre-existing ideas. The interpretation is also influenced by pre-existing ideas. Therefore, after reading the same information different doctors may come to different conclusions about the benefits and costs of a treatment. What is more, after reading the same information presented differently, the same doctor may even come to different conclusions. For example, a treatment with a 34% cardiac event reduction is perceived as more beneficial than a treatment that reduces the absolute risk of cardiac events by 1.4%, even when this actual reduction is identical. Probably because of the higher figure, treatment benefits are perceived as greater when *relative* risk reductions are presented instead of *absolute* risk reductions.

After relevant information has been acquired, the doctor has to make trade-offs. Should one prescribe the highly effective treatment which has some potentially serious side effects and is very costly, or the less effective but also less risky and less expensive treatment? Of course, this trade-off depends on the seriousness of the disease or complaints that have to be treated. Some general observations, however, have been made regarding the relative importance of the various decision criteria in general practice (Denig & Haaijer-Ruskamp, 1995).

In most cases, efficacy, serious side effects, and personal experience are considered to be the most important criteria, closely followed by patient acceptability (i.e. convenience of dosage schedule and administration). The importance of cost, patient wishes, and opinions of colleagues varies a lot depending on the treatment area and on the decision maker. For instance, cost is relatively more important for conditions that are self-limiting and do not necessarily have to be treated with drugs. On the other hand, cost is considered unimportant when treating very serious or acute conditions. The relative importance of cost is also related to the doctor: some are more cost conscious than others. Around one quarter of doctors still do not agree that cost considerations should be taken into account when making prescribing decisions (Denig & Haaijer-Ruskamp, 1995).

The pragmatic approach

Although the analytic model may predict many of the drug choices accurately, it does not necessarily describe what goes on inside a doctor's mind when making a prescribing decision in daily practice. Doctors will make shortcuts in decision-making process for pragmatic reasons. First of all, they will not consider the same trade-offs again and again for frequently occurring situations. In case of repetitive decisions they will develop routine behaviour. Some of these routines may originate from a analytic decision process, but to what extent this is always the case is unknown.

Some routine behaviour is merely copied from peers or superiors without giving it any further thought. Secondly, because of time or cognitive constraints the doctor may settle for a satisfying treatment instead of trying to find the optimal one. Following this strategy, the doctor starts with the first treatment that comes to mind and checks whether this option is good enough; if not, he or she continues searching for a better treatment until a satisfactory one is found. In other words, the treatment options are considered sequentially, and the search can be stopped before all possible options are considered.

Another way of making the decision process easier is to look at the treatment outcomes sequentially instead of balancing risks and benefits simultaneously. For example, a GP starts comparing the different treatments on grounds of efficacy; if one treatment outranks the others that treatment is chosen; only if two or more treatments are equally effective is the next criterion considered. In this case, one outcome does not compensate for another any more. This may lead to prescribing a drug that is superior on the most important outcome, but suboptimal when all relevant outcomes are taken into account.

The intuitive approach

Doctors sometimes resort to simple decision rules based on intuition and personal experience. How this actually works is not really clear. Intuitive thought is rapid and unconscious, and therefore difficult to identify. It has been suggested that intuitive decision makers act upon similarity or pattern recognition and the ability to judge complex patterns without decomposing them into separate features. No trade-off is being made of different options on their separate outcomes. Treatments are chosen because they worked well in previous cases. New problems are solved by adapting solutions that were successful for similar problems.

This type of decision making is not uncommon in medical practice. The more experienced a doctor is, the more he or she will rely on intuition and past experiences. However, this may introduce a considerable bias. Personal observations are usually selective and seldom based on a representative sample of the patient population. On the other hand, it has been argued that a doctor always needs some intuition to decide whether a treatment is optimal for an individual case.

The emotional approach

Decision makers are driven not only by cognitive factors, but also by emotional ones. Emotional motivations can be included in the decision analytic approach, but sometimes decisions are dominated by one feeling. These decisions may even go against the doctor's better (cognitive) judgment, leaving him or her rather uncomfortable about making such a decision (Bradley, 1992). This happens, for instance, when decisions are made to avoid a conflict with a patient or with another doctor, or to please someone.

Dramatic personal experiences may induce subsequent decisions that are dominated by feelings, rather than by cognitive principles. One fatal case can result in dismissing a treatment completely, although the doctor 'knows' that the chances of getting such a result are extremely small and within tolerance. Preventing regret is a further motivation that can dominate prescribing decisions. The feeling of rather being safe than sorry may lead to overprescribing curative and palliative treatments.

This caution factor has been identified as a doctor characteristic that explains prescribing of unnecessary antibiotics. According to doctors who act in this way, too much regret would arise if the condition of the patient did not improve or even deteriorated, because of a wait-and-see attitude, even though they recognize that the 'objective' odds would favour this attitude. There is an opposite reaction when deciding on prescribing preventive treatments to healthy patients: the dominating feeling is then first to do no harm. For example, some doctors, although they believe that oestrogen replacement therapy for menopausal women is beneficial, never prescribe it because of their fear of putting currently healthy women at risk.

Influence of information sources

Regardless of the decision strategy followed, each doctor needs some information about treatments. There are a great number of different sources and routes, the most important ones being pharmaceutical industries, professional sources, government and health insurers, mass media, and patient feedback. None of these sources is completely objective or independent. Each source also may have different niches for doctors.

Some strategies of the pharmaceutical industry, such as advertisements and mailings, are meant to create awareness and prescriber interest for specific drugs. Other activities, such as industry supported books, journals, conferences, and seeding trials, also try to influence the evaluation and adoption of a particular product. The information provided through these channels may be biased. Information about efficacy is often not balanced with the same amount of information about side effects, costs, and contraindications (Ziegler et al., 1995). Although doctors often claim that their final decision to adopt a new drug is not influenced by commercial information, it has been shown that industry-supported activities do influence the decision whether or not to prescribe a new drug.

Professional sources have a limited role in creating awareness and interest for new drugs. The commercial information is often disseminated many months before data are published in peer-reviewed medical journals, and at least a year before it is published in handbooks. However, exchange with professional sources at conferences or personal exchange with colleagues may also create awareness and interest for new drugs. For evaluating the most appropriate role for a drug, most doctors want some information from professional sources. Sometimes this information is only collected to justify the doctors' first judgment of a treatment, but more often they seek objective information about the benefits and costs of a treatment. Some doctors seem to rely more on impersonal sources (publications in books and journals), while others rather rely on personal sources.

The government in the UK and health insurers in some other countries provide drug information as well. In addition to regulatory activities, they publish drug bulletins and reference books to support rational prescribing (see Chapter 1). Governments and other funders of healthcare are also involved in the development and organization of postgraduate education courses though, in the case of the UK, these have not yet been linked specifically to prescribing initiatives such as those described in Chapter 8.

Lately, both government and insurers have focused particularly on promoting cost-effective prescribing. For this reason, they provide information about drug prices, and have actively promoted generic prescribing. Generally speaking, health funders are the main sources of price information. Much of the information about drugs presented to doctors by professional and commercial sources does not highlight drug prices, although with the current initiatives to increase price consciousness of prescribers (see Chapter 7) the most flattering comparisons with main competitors are increasingly presented.

Doctors also get drug information through mass media, as do their patients. Newspapers and television inform both doctors and patients about new developments. Journalists working for these media use scientific journals and press releases from universities and drug companies to select their subjects. Because both the scientific community and the industry communicate their success stories rather than their failures, the mass media present too optimistic a picture of the therapeutic developments (van Trigt, 1995).

Last but not least, doctors learn about drugs from experience. To do so they need feedback from patients. Unfortunately, this information is often incomplete. Patients do not report all possible side effects to their doctor and will seldom volunteer that they did not take their medication as ordered. Furthermore, a patient cannot tell when a treatment was superfluous. If you have received a treatment and got well, you will never know whether the same would have happened without treatment. Despite this uncertainty, most people are inclined to attribute this positive result to the treatment, thus overestimating the usefulness of the treatment.

Dealing with pressures and errors in decision making

Patient pressure

Dealing with the pressure to prescribe from patients means steering a course between the easy option of just giving in and flatly refusing to prescribe without regard to the cost to the doctor–patient relationship. Finding this middle way involves compromise and this is achieved through a process of negotiation between doctor and patient (Bradley, 1994). Doctors sometimes find it difficult to accept this apparently business-derived model of their dealings with patients, but when considered in sociological terms the analogy to negotiation in the world of commerce is remarkably robust. The necessary preconditions of a power gap between the protagonists with one having social control of a resource intensely desired by the other party are completely fulfilled.

Considering the decision of whether or not to prescribe from a negotiation perspective suggests several useful strategies to doctors who may feel themselves under pressure from patients to prescribe. Doctors should recognize, first, that although at times the patient may seem to exert considerable power over them, the ultimate power regarding whether or not a prescription is issued resides with the doctor. Secondly, a deeper understanding of both the doctor's and the patient's negotiating positions is helpful. Thus doctors should consider their tactics not just in terms of whether or not a prescription is issued, but also in terms of whether or not a better, more 'rational' prescription has been issued, or if some ground has been gained in moving the patient toward more 'rational' therapy. The doctor can thereby identify a range of possible and acceptable 'deals' which may still fall short of the ideal of not prescribing.

Considering the patient's position may also provide helpful insights into the scope for reaching a mutually acceptable compromise. Thus, while patients may express very firm and specific expectations from a consultation, there may be a number of possible outcomes of the encounter that would be equally acceptable to them. To do this doctors need to explore more actively with patients their ideas, concerns, and expectations (Pendleton *et al.*, 1984). In so doing, a deeper 'need' underlying an expressed want may often be revealed. For example, a young mother expressing a desire for an antibiotic for her ill child may appear to 'want' an antibiotic but her deeper 'need' may be for a sense of security about her child's future well-being and a feeling of being able to exert some control over the situation.

Finally, reaching a compromise involves generating a number of options that represent a mixture of the desires of doctors and the desires of the patients and choosing between these various options. This can involve some imaginative or lateral thinking. Thus, continuing the example of the mother of the ill child, a promise of a revisit by the doctor and some information about how to spot if things are getting seriously worse might meet the patient's deep felt need for security, such that the expressed 'want' of an antibiotic becomes irrelevant. Any final agreement reached may need to be presented again to the patient in the most favourable possible light in a process described as 'gift wrapping' (Neighbour, 1987).

Other doctors

The key to avoiding the pressure generated by the prescribing of others is communication. A better understanding of the motivation and reasoning behind the prescribing of colleagues makes it easier to agree either to continue with the same prescription or overturn the precedent set previously. What very often makes precedents so difficult to countermand is a lack of insight into how or why the precedent was set in the first place.

There are a variety of mechanisms to encourage communication between colleagues around prescribing issues. One particularly popular and reasonably successful model has involved the development of practice or local formularies and guidelines. It is now recognized that formularies and guidelines are most likely to invoke change in those involved in their development. It has been asserted that it is the process of development that brings about the change rather than the formulary or the guideline itself. Adherence to a formulary or guideline makes prescribing by different doctors in the same practice more consistent and is likely to make individual doctors more internally consistent in their prescribing too. Another increasingly popular strategy is discussion of pharmacotherapy in small peer groups or quality circles.

Precedents set by hospital doctors remain a potential problem, though more recent formulary developments have included attempts to link up hospital and GP formularies. GPs are also becoming more involved in decision making about prescribing policies in hospital. Changes in the relationship between GPs and hospitals in the UK, brought about largely through the purchaser–provider split and the GP fundholding scheme, are beginning to lead to a greater sensitivity of secondary care providers to the requirements of GPs. Among these requirements are that the hospital is not unnecessarily overspecific in its drug recommendations to GPs, nor do they preclude so actively the GP changing the hospital prescription for an essentially similar drug which is in their formulary. Thus where the hospital recommends an NSAID for patient they should ask the primary care doctor to 'prescribe the NSAID of your choice' rather than specifying a particular brand.

Biased information

Doctors are often well aware that printed advertising material and representatives from drug companies are biased in favour of the drug's use (see Chapter 4). Many GPs still believe that these sources are of some use to them. If commercial information sources are used, the messages require careful scrutiny. There should always be questions over whether there is a real need for the drug in general practice.

In the case of written material, doctors should consider exactly what sort of claim is being made for the drug; what sort of evidence is being provided to back up that claim; and what is the quality and trustworthiness of that evidence. Appraising claims made by drug company representatives is potentially more difficult, particularly as the representatives are becoming more and more highly trained in marketing skills. We would suggest that if GPs choose to see representatives at all they should be prepared for the sales pitch and be ready to interrupt it to get the representative focused on a particular question. The key skill with regard to representatives is to keep control of the dialogue and use it to obtain answers to questions rather than allowing representatives to complete their marketing 'spiel'.

GPs must also be on their guard when seeking information elsewhere. Claims made by professional sources also need scrutiny. There is a publication bias towards positive study results, and researchers may overemphasize trivial results in their conclusions. Furthermore, not all information is as independent and reliable as it seems at first glance. Supplements of scientific journals often contain information that was not peer reviewed. Many courses and conferences are supported by parties who have special interests. Again, the pharmaceutical industry is very active here. Sometimes their intentions are clearly visible, but not always. When the financing company is not actively involved in the presentations, it seems that the information presented is unbiased. However, this is not the case if the company has set the agenda and selected only speakers who are in favour of the company's products. The information given may be scientifically sound, but incomplete or unbalanced due to a selection bias. It is very difficult to establish this kind of bias when attending these meetings. One should always be critical and never rely on just one channel of information.

Identifying biased information is not easy, but it is even harder to prevent personal bias. People are always selective when collecting, interpreting, and storing information. To prevent a personal selection bias, it is important not to look only for confirmation of existing beliefs but to keep an open mind towards information that contradicts personal views. When interpreting data most doctors are influenced by the method of presenting and summarizing the results. Vigilance is particularly required when relative reductions or improvements are presented: 50% of almost nothing still remains almost nothing.

Finally, one should be critical of personal observations. People have a tendency to trust confirmatory evidence and distrust negative observations, which are then perceived as being the exception. As a consequence one easily gets the impression that the current routines are adequate and there is no need to change one's behaviour. In addition, when making judgments based on experience one is biased to attribute too much efficacy to the treatment. Therefore, personal experience should be used only in addition to scientific information.

Seeding trials

Conducting 'post-marketing surveillance' trials in general practice is becoming more and more popular. These trials can give the medical community important information about the benefits and risks of drugs in 'real life', provided that the study design is good and the outcomes measured are meaningful. Unfortunately, some trials are mostly of interest to the drug company as a marketing tool. In these so-called seeding trials, GPs are asked to try a new treatment and record just a few—partly subjective—data.

The rewards for participation are often quite generous, but the study will not provide any scientifically interesting results. It is not always easy to determine whether a study design is adequate. One can try to make this judgement oneself, but it is easier to rely on the judgment of a medical ethical committee. This implies that a doctor should only participate in trials that have been approved of by a medical ethical committee. In Holland there is a committee called METOH that evaluates such 'outclinic' trials. After the trial has ended, the participating GP must reconsider the drug's use. One should not automatically adopt the drug in the personal set of drugs because one's experience with the drug during the trial was good. As stated above, personal experience is not enough to make adequate decisions about the value of a drug treatment.

Errors in decision making

Doctors take many shortcuts in their decision making processes. Although the principles used to simplify the decisions are often useful, they can nevertheless lead to certain errors. Routine behaviour is quite appropriate when dealing with frequently occurring situations. One should be aware, though, that routines can become out of date or out of place. It is very hard to change old habits, but routines developed many years ago can become suboptimal and need periodic re-evaluation. A useful method of doing this is to discuss feedback of prescribing data with peers. Such reviewing of prescribing helps to identify routine behaviour that does not live up to current standards.

When evaluating treatments one should force oneself to look at all the relevant benefits and costs. Shortcutting the decision process by looking mainly at the efficacy will lead to overprescribing and unnecessary exposure to risks. Balancing benefits and costs implies that one must consider whether a certain (claimed) benefit justifies (extra) costs. GPs often assume that patients want the most effective drug treatment, but some patients are quite willing to wait and see, or have a less risky or costly alternative, if only they are reassured by the GP (Virji and Britten, 1991). This implies that a GP must discuss different possibilities with patients instead of assuming that these patients want what the doctor thinks is the easiest solution.

One might think that the best decision is a decision based on only cognitive principles, evaluating treatments on their pharmacological and economic outcomes, but this is not the case. It would not be good if patient wishes, clinical intuition, and emotions were omitted entirely from the decisions made in general practice. Good prescribing is not just trying to prescribe effective, safe, and economical treatments, but also treatments that are appropriate for the individual patient. To achieve this, GPs sometimes need to consider the patient's wishes and use past experiences and intuition. However, these motivations should be considered in addition to the cognitive considerations and should not predominate the decision.

References

Abelson, R. P., Levi, A. (1985). Decision making and decision theory. In *The handbook of social psychology*, ed. G. Lindzey, E. Aronson. Random House, New York.

Balint, M., Hunt, J., Joyce, D., Marinker, M., Woodcock, J. (1970). *Treatment or diagnosis: a study of repeat prescriptions in general practice.* Tavistock, London.

Bradley, C. P. (1990). A critical incident study of general practitioners' discomfort arising from prescribing decisions. MD Thesis, University of Dublin, Trinity College, Dublin.

Bradley, C. P. (1991). Decision making and prescribing patterns—a literature review. *Family Practice*, **8**, 276–87.

Bradley, C. P. (1992). Uncomfortable prescribing decisions: a critical incident study. *British Medical Journal*, **304**, 294–6.

Bradley, C. P. (1994). Learning to say no: an exercise in learning to decline inappropriate prescription requests. *Education for General Practice*, **5**, 112–19.

Britten, N. (1994). Patient demand for prescriptions: a view from the other side. *Family Practice*, **11**, 62–6.

Denig, P., Haaijer-Ruskamp, F. M. (1992). Therapeutic decision making of physicians. *Pharmaceutisch Weekblad—Scientific Edition*, **14**, 9–15.

Denig, P. (1994). Drug choice in medical practice. Rationales, routines, and remedies. Dissertation, University of Groningen.

Denig, P., Haaijer-Ruskamp, F. M. (1995). Do physicians take cost into account when making prescribing decisions? *PharmacoEconomics*, **8**, 282–90.

Hall, D. (1980). Prescribing as social exchange. In *Prescribing practice and drug usage*, ed. R. Mapes. Croom Helm, London.

Neighbour, R. (1987). *The inner consultation.* MTP Press, Lancaster.

Pendleton, D., Scofield, T., Tate, P., Havelock, P. (1984). *The consultation: an approach to learning and teaching.* Oxford University Press, Oxford.

Summers, K. H., Szeinbach, S. L. (1993). Formularies: the role of pharmacy-and-therapeutic (P & T) committees. *Clinical Therapeutics*, **15**, 433–41.

Taylor, R. J., Bond, C. M. (1991). Change in the established prescribing habits of general practitioners: an analysis of initial prescriptions in general practice. *British Journal of General Practice*, **41**, 244–8.

van Trigt, A. M. (1995). Making news about medicines. Dissertation, University of Groningen.

Virji, A., Britten, N. (1991). A study of the relationship between patients' attitudes and doctors' prescribing. *Family Practice*, **8**, 314–19.

Ziegler, M. G., Lew, P., Singer, B. C. (1995). The accuracy of drug information from pharmaceutical sales representatives. *Journal of the American Medical Association*, **273**, 1296–8.

CHAPTER SIX

Approaches to rational prescribing

Nicholas Bateman

Expenditure on prescription drugs is increasing in all developed countries at a rate which is disproportionate to the growth in the overall cost of healthcare. This has led governments to focus on prescribing, in an attempt to devise policies which can address this perceived problem (Audit Commission, 1994). The seeming lack of rationality of some prescribing behaviour is an issue which affects developed and developing countries, aspects of which include polypharmacy, the use of unnecessarily expensive therapies, and the inappropriate use of drugs (Hogerzeil, 1995).

A rational prescription can be defined as the issuing of an appropriate drug, at an appropriate dose, for an appropriate period, for a specified therapeutic aim. In the process of consultation a prescription may be used for a number of purposes other than as a treatment for a specific disease. These include as a means of terminating the interview, as reassurance for the patient, and as a bargaining tool. Prescribing statistics suggest that the large majority of consultations in primary care end with a prescription being issued, but the likelihood of this and the profile of drugs prescribed vary substantially between doctors (Wilkin *et al.*, 1987).

Rationality in prescribing requires that a diagnosis is made and that this results in a formal management plan of which the prescription is only one part. In practice, however, the attitude and expectations of patients differ. Whether, or to what extent, it is appropriate that the patient's opinion should be included in an assessment of rational prescribing is ultimately a value judgement, although in overall medical practice taking patients' views into consideration is increasingly regarded as important.

There is a huge difference in the rates of prescribing per head of population in different countries of Europe. In the UK in 1990 around 8 prescriptions per head of population were issued per annum, whereas the figure in France was close to 40. These differences do not reflect differences in morbidity. As a crude number they are also unlikely to be a reflection of differences in rationality either. It is, nevertheless, interesting to note that when the top 20 prescription drugs by volume are evaluated in different European countries the proportion that appear to have clear indications and used with accepted efficacy is high in the UK but low in countries such as Italy, where prescribing volumes are much higher (Garattini and Garattini, 1993).

Reaching a diagnosis in primary care is not always easy, and appropriate, rational, prescribing may be undertaken without a precise pathological diagnosis being available, or necessarily ever being reached. McGavock (1988) has shown the importance of the differences between symptomatic and specific therapies in primary care. For example, a symptomatic therapy would be the use of an analgesic for the management of backache. In contrast, a specific therapy might include treatment for a chronic condition such as hypertension or an acute illness such as a urinary tract infection with an organism of known bacteriological sensitivity. Difficulties in external assessment arise when the same therapy, for example an H_2 antagonist, may be used symptomatically in the treatment of dyspepsia, and specifically to heal ulcers. Similarly, use of antibiotics for a chest infection or a sore throat may be regarded in many cases by the purist as symptomatic therapy since the cause is often viral.

A rational approach to drug choice must start with the establishment of a diagnosis even if this is only provisional. This is followed by the determination of a treatment aim, and then by the selection of an appropriate drug and its prescription at the required dose for an appropriate time period. This approach implies that some prescribed drugs are inherently more appropriate than others. Appropriateness in this context can be considered in terms of efficacy, safety and cost. Unfortunately, precise data on efficacy and safety may not always be available. Independent expert scrutiny of therapies for particular conditions (British Thoracic Society, 1993), particularly when these are linked to a review of published literature (Eccles *et al.*, 1996; North of England Stable Angina Guideline Development Group, 1996; North of England Asthma Guideline Development Group, 1996) will, however, usually offer a professional consensus or evidence-based approach to therapy.

However, precise diagnoses may not always be available at the first consultation, and consensus or evidence-based statements are not available for many conditions seen in primary care. Furthermore, experts do not always agree. Different consensus groups suggest different approaches and the financial impact of advice may not always have been considered. Even when a treatment is accepted as being reasonable, for example the use of angiotensin-converting enzyme (ACE) inhibitors in heart failure, the rationality for use may be questioned by some since the average increase in life expectancy demonstrated in studies using ACE inhibitors is only of the order of 3 months.

Even more difficult is the situation with regard to 'statins', where efficacy has been demonstrated in both primary and secondary prevention (Scandinavian Simvastatin Survival Study Group, 1994: Shepherd *et al.*, 1995), but cost per life saved is of the order of £800000 for primary prevention and nearer £30000 for secondary prevention. Certain sub-groups of higher risk patients, however, have a greater probability of gaining benefits and so a policy of more selective use may achieve much of the benefit at lesser costs than these.

The word 'rational' has itself, therefore, been abused. There is, perhaps inevitably, a tension between the desire for maximum cost benefit and the wish to do the best for individual patients, ignoring the impact of this on the overall health budget. Public health physicians may wish to see the general health of the community improved by a wider study of which drugs are only one part. The patient, on the other hand, will wish to be assured that treatment is most appropriate to his or her personal situation. One reasonable starting point for individual practitioners wishing to consider the rationality of their prescribing is to measure their performance against external indicators. The World Health Organization (WHO, 1993) has produced a list of 12 indicators shown in Box 6.1.

Box 6.1   *Drug use indicators*

Prescribing indicators

1 Average number of drugs per encounter
2 Percentage of drugs prescribed by generic name
3 Percentage of encounters with an antibiotic prescribed
4 Percentage of encounters with an injection prescribed
5 Percentage of drugs prescribed from essential drugs list or formulary

Patient care indicators

6 Average consultation time
7 Average dispensing time
8 Percentage of drugs actually dispensed
9 Percentage of drugs adequately labelled
10 Patient knowledge of correct dosage

Facility indicators

11 Availability of copy of essential drugs list or formulary
12 Availability of key drugs

Number of prescribed drugs

The WHO and (in the UK) the Audit Commission have both highlighted prescribing volume as an indicator which may relate to the quality of medical practice. Such indicators are not always easy to obtain. Thus, the WHO measure, of number of drugs per encounter, would not necessarily be an appropriate marker for a developed country, in which repeat prescribing systems in general practice may operate without a doctor being involved, and where close monitoring of the patients is both possible and desirable. In the UK prescribing volume is more usually expressed as items per head of population, or other appropriate surrogates, for example by population age and gender (Roberts and Harris, 1993).

In the UK the number of prescription items per head is a fairly crude measure, since in a healthcare system which offers the poorer members of society a free prescription, the volume of drugs prescribed which are also available without a prescription in a pharmacy may depend on the socio-economic mix of the practice. This particularly applies to analgesic drugs and childhood remedies such as paracetamol syrup. Nevertheless, practitioners who prescribe more frequently that the average for their own area should review their prescribing policies.

Appropriate starting points for review of prescribing would include the approach to symptomatic therapies such as H_2 antagonists, the frequency of antibiotics prescription for uncomplicated upper respiratory tract infections, and the use of multivitamin preparations.

Generic prescribing

Marketed pharmaceuticals have three names
• the full chemical name (e.g. acetylsalicylic acid)
• a simplified proper 'generic' name (e.g. aspirin)
• a brand name (e.g. Aspro).

A drug has only one generic name, although it may be sold under a variety of brand names. In the UK generic products are made to the same manufacturing standards as their branded equivalents. The government licensing process for generic drugs includes a careful assessment of the manufacturing and formulation processes that they undergo. Generic products are often made by subsidiaries of the companies that market branded drugs.

The use of generic names is conventional in the teaching of therapeutics to medical students in universities. The generic name is devised to inform the practitioner of the general pharmacological group in which the drugs is placed. Examples include the ending 'am' for benzadiazepines (e.g. diazepam, lorazepam), 'olol' for ß-adrenoceptor antagonists (e.g. atenolol, metoprolol, propranolol), and 'pril' for ACE inhibitors (e.g. captopril, enalapril).

In the UK there is, at present, no requirement that generic products exactly match the pattern of absorption of branded products. The removal of the drug from the body depends on its chemical structure and, apart from slow release formulations, not on the pharmaceutical formulation of the compound. Thus, the rate of removal of conventional formulations of generic drugs is exactly the same as that of the branded products.

There are only two situations where formulation of a drug may affect a patient. The first is the rate of absorption of a drug, which in a very limited number of situations may affect concentration-related adverse effects which occur during drug absorption. Where there is a very clear relationship between acute adverse effects and absorption rate, modification of release characteristics may make sufficient difference in plasma concentration profile to cause biological differences. This may apply in some patients using modified release products containing calcium antagonists, in whom flushing and headache occur. These variations are sometimes unpredictable between products and patients. The second is the duration of effect of a drug, particularly in the case of slow release preparations, where the limiting factor in the elimination of the drug from the body is its absorption rate, and hence the absorption rate determines plasma concentration and biological effect. The duration of effect of slow release products may vary, hence brand name prescribing may become necessary.

The issue of generic prescribing is an important one in that it could potentially impinge upon the activities of pharmaceutical companies whose success, and profitability, depend on research innovation. In the UK, however, the profits of the pharmaceutical companies are regulated through the government's Prescription Pricing Regulation Scheme (see Chapter 4), which guarantees companies a return on investment in the UK. Thus, to prescribe by brand name on the basis that this supports local pharmaceutical industries is a mistaken concept, because any shortfall in profit is adjusted for. Similarly, doctors who prescribe so-called 'branded' generics in the belief that they are cheaper than other generic drugs misunderstand the pricing structure in the UK. Drug tariff prices are adjusted on a regular basis and the prices of such compounds can be adjusted, without the prescriber necessarily being aware that this has happened.

In practice, therefore, apart from a small number of slow release preparations and some biological products, for example influenza vaccines, for which there is no generic substitute, generic prescribing is both rational and cost effective. Nevertheless, practitioners will continue to be subject to propaganda on this issue. Examples include attacks on the use of generic inhalers in asthma (Pearson *et al.*, 1994) and the use of generic prescribing in epilepsy (Crawford *et al.*, 1996). The former allegation of generic inequivalents for inhalers is clearly flawed (Smith and Bateman, 1995) and the Crawford study, used leading questions in epileptic patients and so is scientifically flawed. Both papers illustrate the need to communicate prescribing decisions with patients and, ideally, to maintain prescribing supplies from the same manufacturing source.

Most GPs have seen generic prescribing as an important way in which they can limit prescribing expenditure, at no cost to patient care (Eccles *et al.*, 1996). The fact that most GP computing systems now contain a generic option for prescribing means that this good practice, and economic sense, is readily available in primary care.

Ineffective prescribing

All pharmaceutical products marked in the UK are licensed on the basis of safety and efficacy. Nevertheless, there is evidence that some drugs are frequently prescribed inappropriately by some prescribers. Thus, a consensus group of GPs considered that cerebral vasodilators, which have no demonstrable effect in dementia, and peripheral vasodilators, for which evidence of significant improvement in outcome in astherosclerosis is weak, should not normally be prescribed in primary care (Bateman *et al.*, 1996).

Similarly, appetite suppressants produce short term weight reduction, but evidence that long term weight reduction is maintained on stopping therapy is poor. The vast majority of patients regain any weight they have lost. These drugs show marked cyclical prescribing which varies with the season of the year (Thomas and Campbell, 1996), indicating that patient demand is likely to be a significant driving force for prescribing rather than clinical need. A number of other drug groups are of doubtful efficacy, including multivitamin preparations, antitussives, and oral decongestants.

Inappropriate prescribing

In this context inappropriate prescribing refers to the administration of a prescription drug in situations where this is not strictly necessary. In primary care the use of a prescription to terminate a consultation is a well-recognized technique, which can readily lead to inappropriate prescribing. The prescription may have some logic, for example an antibiotic for a respiratory tract infection; or it may be a pseudo-placebo, for example the use of a multivitamin preparation. Questions that the prescriber needs to consider are: firstly, whether this is a condition for which a prescription drug is indicated; and, secondly, what is the aim of therapy. Only if these two questions can be answered should a drug be prescribed, particularly since the issuing of a prescription will reinforce the belief in the patient that future presentations for similar problems require drug therapy.

The management of upper respiratory tract infections is an area which causes considerable controversy. While it is recognized that for most patients with a sore throat or cough a viral origin to the condition is highly likely, antibiotics are still frequently prescribed. This is an area where patient demand and expectation is often a factor and, while scientific data suggests that antibiotics are in general unnecessary, prescribing is a well-established patterns expected by patients. Even here, however, if counselling on the lack of need for an antibiotic is unsuccessful a rational drug choice can be made on the basis of the likely organism, if a bacterial infection were present. A short course of the relatively cheap amoxycillin is more appropriate than a more expensive broader spectrum agent. Antibiotic resistance in the community relating to excess antibiotic prescribing should be a concern to all prescribers. Countries with high antibiotic prescribing rates, such as France and Spain, have much higher rates of antibiotic resistance than the UK.

Appropriate prescribing rates

It is difficult to define clearly the level of 'necessary' prescribing in an individual practice. Local norms may offer some guidance, for example average prescribing rates in a health authority area. Summary comparative data may be quite difficult to obtain, although PACT data in England provides some local (Health Authority) comparator data (see Chapter 8). Levels of prescribing in different Health Authorities do vary widely. Thus data on appetite suppressant prescribing shows a wide range in prescribing per head of population in different practices. At Health Authority level, rates of use of appetite suppressants in the nine former Family Health Services Authorities in the former UK Northern Region varied approximately twofold. Although the trend was for a reduction in the use of these agents, this variation persisted between 1989 and 1994, with the highest prescribing area prescribing an average twice as much as the lowest prescriber in the area (Thomas and Campbell, 1996). Similarly, larger variation can be shown in individual practices for antiulcer drugs, antiasthma drugs, and cardiovascular preparations (Roberts and Bateman, 1994a,b; 1995).

Inappropriate management of adverse effects

All prescription drugs cause adverse effects, although the frequency and type of adverse effects obviously vary. It is convenient to consider these adverse effects as usually either primarily due to the pharmacology of the drug (type A effects) or unrelated to the primary pharmacology, and therefore unpredictable (type B effects). Type A effects include, for example, tiredness with beta blockers, dry mouth with anticholinergics, sedation with anxiolytics, constipation with opiates, and dyspepsia with NSAIDs. Rather than consider alternative therapies, clinicians will sometimes respond to these adverse effects by prescribing an additional drug to treat the symptoms of the first. This in turn will have its own pattern of adverse effects.

An example of where combination prescribing can have significant cost implications is the present controversy over the use of concommitent antiulcer therapy with NSAID agents. The risk of gastrointestinal bleeding increases with age (Somerville *et al.*, 1986) and so it is the elderly who have become the target of industry attempts to persuade prescribers to provide routine therapy with antiulcer preparations, for example misoprostol or H_2 antagonists, when prescribing a NSAID. The temptation is to prescribe two drugs, rather than to review the appropriateness of a NSAID even thought the use of simple analgesics should be the primary aim in the elderly (Bateman and Kennedy, 1995). The situation is further complicated by conflicting pharmaco-economic analyses of prescribing ulcer prophylaxis that have been published (Maiden and Madhok, 1995). It is this author's view that prophylaxis is generally not appropriate without a clear history of a proven peptic ulcer, or other risk factor.

Rationalizing prescription length

In general practice, approximately 65% of prescriptions are 'repeats', thus indicating these are long term therapies. Repeat prescriptions account for approximately 75% of cost of prescription drugs (Audit Commission, 1994). The repeat prescribing system is a potential cause of three types of waste. These are:

* waste arising from inappropriate continuation of the therapy
* excessive prescribing of repeat 'as required' prescriptions
* waste arising from prescriptions of varying duration and quantity for different therapies in the same patient.

Appropriate review of the need for repeat prescriptions is important. This is often most difficult when patients are under the care of both primary and secondary sectors. In this situation, the need for an individual therapy is often assumed by each parties as being established by the other. Here communication, in both directions is important, and it is necessary to review the indications for any therapy given on a repeat basis at regular intervals, for example every 6 or 12 months.

If patients are prescribed therapies for different treatment intervals this can also lead to waste. For example a combined prescribing for 28 and 31 day courses of two different drugs results, over a 12 month period, in an excess supply of 36 days' treatment. It is, therefore, important that repeat prescribing policies are drawn up within individual practices to avoid such potential problems. Difficulties also arise when a combination of 'as required' and regular prescriptions are given, and it is important to educate patients, perhaps with the help of community pharmacists, to request appropriate supplies to avoid wastage. These details seem superficially minor, but can lead to considerable cost savings since, for example, an irregular prescribing duration pattern will result in a 10% wastage in a drug given to a 31 day as opposed to a 28 day period. 10% of NHS drug costs in primary care is over £350 million.

So much of GP prescribing is for repeat medications that interventions to modify prescribing behaviour of acute medications may not appear to influence the pattern of prescribing in a practice in the short term. It is, however, also necessary to consider acute prescribing, and again the duration of acute, short term prescriptions is an appropriate area for prescribing rationality. For example, the duration of antibiotic prescribing should be for as short a period as necessary. Three day courses of antibiotics for urinary tract infections and 5 day courses for chest infections will generally be adequate for most adults. On the other hand, most antidepressant therapies take 3–4 months to become effective. If a high proportion of patients only receive one prescription in any course of treatment then a review of diagnostic criteria of depression used by that doctor would seem advisable.

Habituation

A number of drugs cause dependence, the most important being benzodiazepines and opiates. It is therefore very important to avoid development of dependence by careful attention to the initial prescribing of drugs in these categories. Short courses of hypnotic drugs should be used, and patients should be warned that if they have been on a short course of hypnotic drugs they are likely to suffer withdrawal insomnia when therapy is stopped.

Although opiate dependence is unlikely in the management of acute severe pain, for example postoperatively in hospital, use of opiates for chronic, non-malignant pain is more difficult. Some patients escalate their dosage rapidly and become dependent, whereas others seem able to obtain good relief from low doses. The issue here is the management of the dosing regimen by the practitioner, the avoidance of duplicate prescribing, or shortened repeat prescribing intervals within the practice, and awareness of the risk of development of dependence.

Pharmaceutical formulation

The pharmaceutical industry has been very successful in developing sophisticated drug delivery systems. These include slow release products, sublingual products, and patch formulations. Each of these routes of drug administration has an important place in therapy. Nevertheless, there is a temptation to over-engineer pharmaceutical products. These products are not only more expensive, but often offer no real therapeutic advantage to the patient. Claims of improvements in compliance for such products are also often overstated.

One example of a modified release product which was inappropriate was that of the modified release product indomethacin which released the drug by osmosis (Osmosin). This product resulted in a high incidence of adverse effects because of the local actions of indomethacin on the small bowel.

An appropriate use of a slow release formulation is to allow simpler dosing regimens for drugs with short half-lives, where regular dosing with a standard preparation would be impractical. Two good examples of this are slow release theophylline preparations and slow release morphine. In both cases, however, dose titration is necessary. A further appropriate use of a modified release preparation is in situations where the absorption profile of the parent drug results in significant adverse effects. Examples of this are few, but one is to alter the rate of absorption of levodopa in patients with Parkinson's disease, where, on rare occasions, acute dyskinetic problems may result from the sharp rise in drug concentration during the absorption phase, particularly in patients who have been receiving levodopa for some years and have developed the 'on–off' syndrome. This can be reduced by the use of a slow release product. In the case of levodopa, which is also relatively short acting, a slow release preparation also results in a longer duration of clinical efficacy. This is only appropriate, however, for a minority of patients with Parkinson's disease, and should not be considered as rational first line therapy.

Slow release formulations are not appropriate for drugs with very long half-lives. Thus, slow release preparations of amitriptyline (which has a half-life of 10–24 hours and an active metabolite nortriptyline with a half-life of 20–30 hours) are unnecessary, make no therapeutic sense, and are expensive.

Sublingual preparations, which are absorbed across the buccal mucosa, avoid being metabolized at first pass through the liver, and thus may be of benefit for drugs that undergo extensive first-pass metabolism. This may be useful in acute situations, for example sublingual nitrate in patients with acute myocardial ischaemia, but makes little sense in the chronic situation, where a higher oral dose can be provided at a far cheaper cost with no difference in clinical outcome.

Claims that slow release preparations improve compliance (or, as it is now more correctly termed, adherence) because they have to be taken less often, are difficult to substantiate. In practice, adherence only tends to be a significant issue when patients have to take drugs more than twice a day, and where there is no acute symptomatic benefit to the individual drugs, for example in the management of hypertension.

Transdermal (patch) formulations also avoid first-pass metabolism and, theoretically, can offer a steady slow input of drug into the blood stream, producing an effect which is similar to a constant intravenous infusion. These products are, however, extremely expensive and, offer few clinical benefits. An example of where the transdermal route is of benefit is the use of the analgesic fentanyl, in patients with terminal illness who cannot swallow. The routine use of oestrogen patches for hormone replacement therapy is, on the other hand, far more difficult to defend on a cost–benefit basis. They should be reserved for the small minority of women who develop adverse effects with oral oestrogen that are related to plasma concentration.

Efficacy

Pharmaceutical products are licensed for specific indications, for which evidence of efficacy is obtained from controlled clinical trials. Prior to marketing such clinical trials have usually only been done on a few hundred, or at most a few thousand, patients. It is thus rare for the appropriate clinical niche of a drug to be established at an early stage after marketing. To establish comparative efficacy between drugs in the same therapeutic area requires much more detailed studies, and these need to involve many more patients. In addition, it is much easier to establish comparative efficacy for a surrogate marker, for example a change in blood pressure, than for the more clinically relevant marker, which in hypertension would be the incidence of stroke or myocardial infarction. Construction of clinical comparisons are complex, because individual patients may vary in their responsiveness to different agents, and vary in their susceptibility to as adverse effects.

An example of the complexity of comparative efficacy studies is that of the use of antidepressant drugs. Older tricyclic antidepressants have a well-documented list of adverse effects, and are toxic in overdose. Newer anti-depressants of the selective serotonin reuptake inhibitor (SSRI) class have a different profile of adverse effects, although interestingly the overall incidence of these seems close to that experienced with tricyclics (Song *et al.*, 1993; MacDonald *et al.*, 1996). In overdose, however, they are less toxic (Henry *et al.*, 1995). Direct comparative efficacy studies cannot be readily performed and epidemiological studies are necessary. These suggest that the suicide rate in patients themselves taking SSRIs may be similar to that of patients prescribed tricyclic antidepressants (Jick *et al.*, 1995; Edwards, 1995). The potential advantage of being safer in overdose does not necessarily produce a better clinical outcome (Song *et al.*, 1993). This is one of the more obvious examples of where a newer drug may have theoretical advantages over an older product, but where detailed evaluation is required to document the rational choice, which for antidepressants might be the compromise of lofepramine. In practice it seems likely that many patients are prescribed relatively low doses of antidepressants, raising questions on diagnosis on necessity for drug therapy (Kendrick, 1996).

The toxicity profile itself can be used to underpin rational prescribing. An example of this is the toxicity profile of NSAIDs. In epidemiological studies these can be shown to have different rates of peptic ulceration associated with them. Thus ibuprofen appears to have the safest adverse reaction profile when serious adverse effects on the gastrointestinal tract are considered, drugs such as naproxen and diclofenac have intermediate toxicity, and azapropazone and piroxicam are the most toxic. Piroxicam and azapropazone do not, therefore, appear to be appropriate NSAIDs to use as first line therapy (Bateman, 1994).

Monitoring rational approaches

The prescriber who is using a rational approach to prescribing will wish to monitor this. The monitoring system will therefore be likely to include measures in at least four areas. These would include generic prescribing, low use of inappropriate or ineffective therapies, evidence that a range of drugs is used, and evidence that the duration of therapy of drugs such as benzodiazepine hypnotics is appropriate. One such system for monitoring prescribing quality using prescription data has been published, and used to monitor prescribing in an NHS region (Northern and Yorkshire) since 1993 (Bateman *et al.*, 1996). The criteria against which prescribing is measured are shown in Box 6.2.

Techniques to aid rational prescribing

There are a number of simple techniques that practitioners can adopt to assist in their search for rational prescribing practice. These include the use of formularies. These may be externally derived, but periodically will be of more practical value if some of the policies adopted are as a result of practice reviews, with peer audit from colleagues. These reviews could involve the local community pharmacist or health authority prescribing adviser.

Box 6.2 *Criteria of prescribing quality (from Bateman et al., 1996)*

Generic prescribing

Drug choice within a therapeutic group

Frusemide and bendrofluazide as percentage of diuretics

Atenolol and prop ranolol as percentage of beta-blockers

Amitriptyline, dothiepin, imipramine and lofepramine as percentage of antidepressants

Twelve antibacterials as percentage of antibiotic prescribing

Diclofenac, ibuprofen, indomethacin, and naproxen as percentage of NSAIDs

Drugs of limited clinical value

Diuretic-potassium combinations

Cerebral and peripheral vasodilators

Compound antidepressants

Appetite suppressants

Topical NSAIDs

Prescribing volume

Benzodiazepines

Lorazepam

Education in therapeutics is a second approach, and a number of universities now offer postgraduate courses in therapeutics targeted at general practice. Education may be done in other ways, one example being the Nelson project in New Zealand, in which case studies are used to encourage rational prescribing (Ferguson *et al.*, 1995). Finally, the potential for computer aided prescribing advice at the point of consultation, such as the Dutch Prescriptor system and its UK equivalent, PRODIGY, is under development (see Chapter 9).

Most doctors would agree that improvement in quality of care of their patients is a laudable aim. Improvements in prescribing behaviour will help to address this. The development of rational approaches to prescribing in primary care is fundamental to this process.

References

Audit Commission (1994). *A prescription for improvement—towards more rational prescribing in general practice.* Audit Commission, London.

Bateman, D. N. (1994). NSAIDs: time to re-evaluate gut toxicity. *Lancet*, **343**, 1051–2.

Bateman, D. N., Eccles, M., Campbell, M., Soutter, J., Roberts, S. J., Smith, J. M. (1996). Setting standards of prescribing performance in primary care: use of a consensus group of general practitioners and application of standards to practices in the north of England. *British Journal of General Practice*, **46**, 20–5.

Bateman, D. N., Kennedy, J. G. (1995). Non-steroidal anti-inflammatory drugs and elderly patients. *British Medical Journal*, **310**, 817–18.

British Thoracic Society (1993). Guidelines on the management of asthma. *Thorax*, **48**, (Suppl) S1–S24.

Crawford, P., Hall, W. H., Chappel, B., Collings, J., Stewart, A. (1996). Generic prescribing for epilepsy. Is it safe? *Seizure*, **5**, 1–5.

Eccles, M., Clapp, Z., Grimshaw, J., Adams, P. C., Higgins, B., Purves, I., Russell, I. (1996). North of England evidence based guidelines development projects: methods of guideline development. *British Medical Journal*, **312**, 760–2.

Eccles, M. P., Soutter, J., Bateman, D. N., Campbell, M., Smith, J. M. (1996). Influences on prescribing in non-fundholding general practices. *British Journal of General Practice*, **46**, 287–90.

Edwards, J. G. (1995). Suicide and antidepressants. *British Medical Journal*, **310**, 205–6.

Ferguson, R. I., Salmond, C. E., Maling, T. J. B. (1995). The Nelson Prescribing Project—A programmed intervention in General Practice in New Zealand. *PharmacoEconomics*, **7**, 555–61.

Garattini, S., Garattini, L. (1993). Pharmaceutical prescription in four European countries. *Lancet*, **342**, 1191–2.

Henry, J. A., Alexander, C. A., Sener, E. K. (1995). Relative mortality from overdose of antidepressants. *British Medical Journal*, **310**, 221–4.

Hogerzeil, H. V. (1995). Promoting rational prescribing: an international perspective, *British Journal of Clinical Pharmacology*, **39**, 1–6.

Jick, S. S., Dean, A. D., Jick, H. (1995). Antidepressants and suicide. *British Medical Journal*, **310**, 215–18.

Kendrick, T. (1996). Prescribing antidepressants in general practice. *British Medical Journal*, **313**, 829–30.

MacDonald, T. M., McMahon, A. D., Reid, I. C., Fenton, G. W., McDevitt, D. G. (1996). Antidepressant drug use in primary care: a record linkage study in Tayside, Scotland. *British Medical Journal*, **313**, 860–1.

McGavock, H. (1988). Some patterns of prescribing by urban general practitioners. *British Medical Journal*, **296**, 900–2.

Maiden, N., Madhok, R. (1995). Misoprostol in patients taking non-steriodal anti-inflammatory drugs. *British Medical Journal*, **311**, 1518–19.

North of England Stable Angina Guideline Development Group (1996). North of England evidence based guidelines development project: summary version of evidence based guideline for the primary care management of stable angina. *British Medical Journal*, **312**, 827–32.

North of England Asthma Guideline Development Group (1996). North of England evidence based guidelines development project: summary version of evidence based guideline for the primary care management of asthma in adults. *British Medical Journal*, **312**, 762–6.

Pearson, M., Lewis, R., Watson, J., Ayres, J., Ibbotson, G., Ryan, D., Flynn, D., Williams, J. (1994). Generic inhalers for asthma. *British Medical Journal*, **309**, 1440.

Roberts, S. J., Bateman, D. N. (1995). Prescribing of antacids and ulcer-healing drugs in primary care in the north of England. *Alimentary and Pharmacological Therapy*, **9**, 137–43.

Roberts, S. J., Bateman, D. N. (1994a). Which patients are prescribed inhaled anti-asthma drugs? *Thorax*, **49**, 1090–5.

Roberts, S. J., Bateman, D. N. (1994b). The use of nitrates, calcium channel blockers and ACE inhibitors in primary care in the Northern Region: a pharmacoepidemiological study. *British Journal of Clinical Pharmacology*, **38**, 489–97.

Roberts, S. J., Harris, C. M. (1993). Age, sex and temporary resident originated prescribing units (ASTRO-PUs) new weightings for analysing prescribing of general practice in England. *British Medical Journal*, **307**, 485–8.

Scandinavian Simvastatin Survival Study Group (1994). Randomised trial of cholesterol lowering in 4444 patients with coronary heart disease: the Scandinavian Simvastatin Survival Study (4S). *Lancet*, **344**, 1383–9.

Shepherd, J., Cobbe, S. M., Ford, I., Isles, C. G., Lorimer, A. R., MacFarlane, P. W., McKillop, J. H., Packard, C. J. (1995). Prevention of coronary heart disease with pravastatin in men with hypercholesterolemia. *New England Journal of Medicine*, **333**, 1301–7.

Smith, J. M., Bateman, D. N. (1995). Treating asthma. *British Medical Journal*, **310**, 254.

Somerville, K., Faulkner, G., Langman, M. (1986). Non-steroidal anti-inflammatory drugs and bleeding peptic ulcer. *Lancet* **1**: 462–4.

Song, F., Freemantle, N., Sheldon, T. A., House, A., Watson, P., Long, A., Mason, J. (1993). Selective serotonin reuptake inhibitors: meta-analysis of efficacy and acceptability. *British Medical Journal*, **306**, 683–7.

Thomas, S. H. L., Campbell, M. (1996). Utilization of appetite suppressants in England: A putative indicator of poor prescribing practice. *Pharmacoepidemiology and Drug Safety*, **5**, 237–46.

Wilkin, D., Hallam, L., Leavey, R., Metcalfe, D. (1987). Patterns of care. In *Anatomy of urban general practice*, Chapter 7. Tavistock, London.

WHO (1993) *How to investigate drug use in health facilities: selected drug use indicators*. WHO/DAP/93. 1, World Health Organization, Geneva.

CHAPTER SEVEN

Health economics and prescribing

Alan Earl-Slater

Primary healthcare professionals have more reason to be interested in health economics than many currently appreciate. Anyone working to improve patient wellbeing within the restrictions incurred by limited resources (time, skills, knowledge, and funds) can benefit from an understanding of health economics. The fundamental principles addressed using health economic tools and techniques, i.e. that resources are limited and that this forces choices between different courses of actions with different costs and benefits flowing from them, are not new but have always been part and parcel of medical practice. What health economics offers is a rational, explicit, and accountable way of making the decisions that have to be made.

As discussed in the preceding chapter, rational prescribing is based on a balance between safety, efficacy, appropriateness, and cost. While traditionally more attention has, perhaps, been focused on the technical medical issues of safety and efficacy, the current emphasis on the finite nature of resources has brought two other issues to prominence. Firstly, what are the costs involved in achieving the effects of healthcare intervention?; and secondly, is there room for improvement? These two questions can be compacted into what is called 'the search for value for money' in healthcare. This search is the core driving force behind the more explicit use of economics in healthcare.

Types of economic assessment of healthcare interventions

There are a variety of ways to evaluate any healthcare intervention. Exactly which method of assessment is chosen depends on the question asked and what information is needed. To know which tool to then use, requires an appreciation of the strengths and weaknesses of the various tools.

Fig. 7.1 *The assessment decision tree*

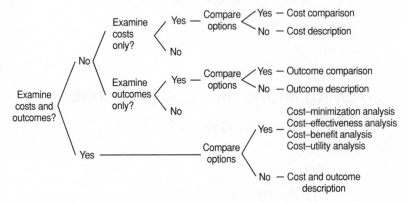

Figure 7.1 is a decision tree representing different types of economic assessment with a variety of uses:

- it signals the differences between various types of assessment
- it shows where there are similarities
- it serves to outline some of the limitations of each type of assessment
- the decision tree in itself can serve as a checklist to ensure the appropriate form of assessment is chosen.

By progressing along the appropriate branches (reading from left to right) one can trace out what has to be done in order to perform a certain type of assessment. For example to perform a cost-comparison analysis requires the comparison of the costs of at least two different possible healthcare interventions. The decision tree can also be used as a checklist to appraise a health economic evaluation by reading from right to left. Thus, if a claim is being made that an outcome-comparison is the endpoint, then reading right to left from the outcome-comparison endpoint of Fig. 7.1, shows that this particular method of assessment involves comparing the outcomes of more than one possible healthcare intervention.

The first stage in the decision tree asks if one is examining costs and consequences of healthcare intervention. If the interest lies in just the outcomes of a healthcare decision, then the answer to the first question 'Examine costs and outcomes? is no. Interest only in comparing outcomes achievable under treatment regimen A versus treatment regimen B then leads to an *outcome comparison*. If the GP is only interested in the outcomes from regimen A then the method to chose is an *outcome description*.

Increasingly, the primary care professional is faced with more than one healthcare option: option A versus option B, for example. If one is only interested in the costs involved in either of the two courses of action, A or B, then under this scenario the appropriate analysis to undertake is a *cost comparison of A versus B*. On the other hand if one is only interested in the outcomes possible from either of the two courses of action then under this scenario the appropriate method of analysis is technically called an *outcome comparison of A versus B*.

For analysis of costs and outcomes of different possible courses of healthcare action, four different types of assessment are available:
• cost-minimization analysis
• cost-effectiveness analysis
• cost–benefit analysis
• cost-utility analysis.

These four types of analysis have important differences. Table 7.1 shows the similarities and differences between the four methods of assessment. The essential difference between the four types of assessment lie in the area of the *outcomes*. There are two dimensions to the outcomes: first the unit of measurement of the outcomes; second, if the outcomes are *a priori* assumed to be worthwhile.

Table 7.1 *Comparing costs and consequences of policy*

Type of analysis	Denominator for costs	Consequences
Cost-minimization	£	Identical in all important respects Measured (by assumption or calculus) Plays no further part in assessment Assumed worthwhile
Cost-effectiveness	£	Single or mixed effects achieved to different degrees Measured in natural units[a] Assumed worthwhile
Cost–benefit	£	Single or mixed effects Measured in £ Not *a priori* assumed worthwhile
Cost-utility	£	Single or mixed effects Measured in units of utility Not *a priori* assumed worthwhile

[a] *Such as blood pressure, temperature, lumbar flexion, visual acuity, degree of infection.*

Cost-minimization analysis

If, for example, drug A and drug B would achieve the same outcomes, or if the outcomes are not significantly different, then the appropriate type of analysis would be a *cost-minimization analysis*. Hence, if treatment regimen A costs less than B, the GP would opt for treatment regime A and minimize the costs of achieving the same amount of outcomes. Three assumptions exist for cost-minimization analysis:

- there is a fundamental *a priori* assumption that the outcomes from the interventions are worthwhile
- that multiple or single outcomes from healthcare intervention are captured and are to all intents and purposes the same
- that all the outcomes from healthcare intervention can be measured in comparable units—the actual units of measurement are irrelevant.

Cost-effectiveness analysis

The second form of economic analysis in Table 7.1 is called *cost-effectiveness analysis.* The term 'cost-effectiveness' has come to be used very loosely as part of everyday language in the healthcare arena, often incorrectly with respect to its proper technical health economic meaning. Strictly speaking, *cost-effectiveness analysis* involves the comparison of costs and outcomes of two or more possible interventions when the costs are in monetary units and the outcomes or effects are in 'natural units'. Natural units include such measures as years of life saved, cholesterol level, visual acuity, body temperature, lumbar flexion, number of inoculations, incidence of the ill-health condition, prevalence of the condition, and more generally mortality or morbidity rates.

Cost-effectiveness analysis is most useful where the costs of possible interventions may differ and the effects may also differ in magnitude (but are measured in the same natural units). For example suppose the hospital operation A costs £13500 for the electrophysiology stimulation in treatment of ventricular arrhythmias. Suppose that the hospital intervention saves the lives of 8 out of 10 patients. The alternative healthcare intervention is a course of drug B at a cost of £750, and drug intervention is successful in the same terms, i.e. lives saved, in 6 out of 10 patients.

The critical calculation of interest in cost-effectiveness analysis is the costs per unit effect. What is the value for money from deciding to go for intervention A or B? In this example the cost per unit effect is the cost per life year saved. A course of hospital electrophysiology stimulation costs £1687.50 (£13500/0.8) per life saved; for primary care drug intervention a course costs £1250 (£750/0.6) per life saved. On the basis of this evidence then drug intervention in primary care is *more cost-effective* than hospital electrophysiology stimulation in the treatment of ventricular arrhythmias.

Cost-effectiveness analysis differs significantly from *cost analysis* and from *outcomes analysis.* For example, if one was only interested in the costs of healthcare intervention A or B above then, on the data presented above, one would go for the drug treatment route at a cost of £750 per patient course: this is *cost analysis.* On the other hand if one was only interested in the outcomes of intervention A or B, the number of lives saved in this instance, then one would go for hospital intervention as it saves 80% of lives whereas the drug intervention saves only 60%; this is on the basis of *outcome analysis.*

Two principles of cost-effectiveness analysis are:
- there is an *a priori* assumption that the outcomes from the interventions are beneficial
- that there can be multiple outcomes from intervention and one need not be restricted to looking at single outcomes from healthcare intervention.

The difficulty, however, is how to reconcile any package of outcomes if the outcomes are in mixed natural units, such as a basket of outcomes of interest involving lives saved, blood pressure, and cholesterol levels from healthcare intervention. One attempted solution would be to recalculate the packages of outcomes into a single common unit of measurement: an index number. Another possible solution is for an explicit decision to be made on the most important clinical outcome and just use that as the unit of outcome measurement. In the example above, the lives saved is probably the most important endpoint or outcome in the treatment of ventricular arrhythmias. An intermediate position to pull together the packages of outcomes is to weigh the various outcomes from each intervention and determine an index of weighted natural outcomes.

Cost–benefit analysis

The distinguishing characteristics of cost–benefit analysis are:
- there can be more than one outcome
- the outcome(s) are calculated in monetary terms
- the outcomes are not *a priori* assumed to be worthwhile.

There are inherent difficulties in calculating outcomes in money terms; for example, how does one accurately calculate the value of lives saved in the treatment of ventricular arrhythmias in money terms? One possible procedure is to determine what people are willing to pay for certain sets of outcomes and use these willingness to pay factors as the relevant monetary units. Willingness to pay is, however, inextricably linked up with the ability to pay: those who can afford to pay more for certain outcomes may yield a greater willingness to pay for certain outcomes.

If outcomes can be calculated in money terms, cost–benefit analysis is the appropriate form of analysis to use but is actually not often used in healthcare.

Cost-utility analysis

The distinguishing characteristics of cost-utility analysis are:
- the outcomes are calculated in terms of utility or subjective value
- the outcomes are not *a priori* assumed worthwhile
- the outcomes can be singular or multiple.

One way to determine the outcomes in utility terms is to use the concept of the quality adjusted life year (QALY). A QALY aims to capture the fact that healthcare intervention affects the quality of the patient's life and the life expectancy or the length of that life. By dividing the total cost by the total QALY of each possible course of intervention, one can determine the cost per unit QALY gained. The choice then would be to go for the healthcare intervention that offers the lowest cost per unit QALY gained. The main difficulty with QALY is that the quality of life aspect is sensitive to how it is captured. The quality of life (QoL) element can vary, so the QALY outcome unit depends heavily on the QoL.

Other ways are to determine the impact of healthcare intervention by using QoL questionnaires. However, healthcare aims to affect the length of life, not just the quality of life.

If outcomes can be calculated in terms of utility then cost-utility analysis is the appropriate form of analysis to use. Like any other outcome measure the QALY has been greeted with mixture of enthusiasm, scepticism, confusion, and consternation.

The measurement of outcomes

How one identifies and measures health (life expectancy and quality of life) and the impacts that primary healthcare professionals make on peoples' lives is an increasingly important part of healthcare. There is a growing literature on outcomes in healthcare and the purpose of this section is to give an introduction to some of the issues in identifying, measuring and valuing healthcare impact.

Quality of life measures

One of the most common reasons for measuring health then is to measure performance of healthcare intervention, e.g. drugs, surgery, counselling. This is usually with a view to securing better value for money in healthcare. The job of measuring outcomes can be approached by splitting it into four component measures of health:

- clinical
- physical
- psychological
- social.

Figure 7.2 illustrates the health measurement pyramid. At the top of the pyramid is a collection of health measures called *health indices*. Indices are deduced from *health profiles* which are themselves made up of some or all of the four components at the bottom of the pyramid: clinical, physical, psychological and social measures of health. A *health profile* then is a collection of details or perceptions about the person's health whereas *health indices* are summary figures of the person's health or perceived health status.

Moving along the bottom of the pyramid from left to right the components become more subjective in measurement, whereas moving from right to left the components become more objective.

The pyramid can be used for a variety of purposes:

Fig. 7.2 *The health measurement pyramid*

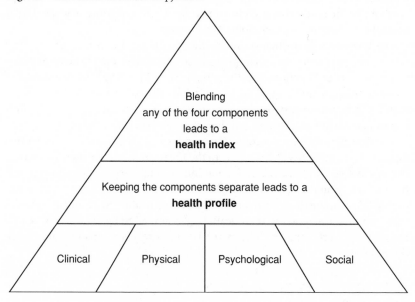

- it helps discern differences between health measurements
- it can be used to see similarities between measures of health
- it will serve to outline some of the limitations of each type of measurement of health, e.g. some indices only include clinical measures of health
- it can serve as a useful checklist for any measure of health
- it can be used as a cognitive map to help remember the first four uses.

The usefulness of any measure of health, however, turns on a variety of points:
- the *question* at hand
- the *perspective* of the analysts
- the *validity* of the measurement (i.e. does it measure what it alleges to measure)
- the *reliability* of the measurement (i.e. the stability or consistency in the results if the measurement tool is used again).

Health profiles try to build up a picture of the health of the patient. One such measure is the Nottingham Health Profile (NHP), first developed in the 1970s. The NHP is designed to be a measure of perceived health of the patient and includes points on physical mobility, pain, energy, sleep, social isolation, and emotional reactions. The Sickness Impact Profile (SIP), like the NHP, includes detail on a societal dimension of health. The scope of the SIP includes alertness behaviour, body movement/body care, eating, emotional behaviour, mobility, home management, sleep and rest, recreation and pastimes, ambulation, work. and social interaction. Many other health profile measurements, e.g., SBQOL, and SF36 exist. The titles of some health measures can unfortunately be deceptive: for instance the General Well-being Index is not a measure of general well-being, but a measure of psychological well-being.

The Karnofsky performance index (KPI) started out as a measure of ward nursing requirements but was improved and adapted for the purposes of measuring the physical functioning of the patient. The KPI is determined by means of a questionnaire consisting of 10 questions for the patient and it takes only a matter of a minute or two to complete. Thus health indices need not have all four components (clinical, physical, psychological, and social) in their base.

The Rosser *et al.* index is a collection of indices in a matrix and combines two aspects of life: disability and distress. In the Rosser *et al.* matrix there exists four degrees of distress (A, B, C, and D) and initially eight levels of disability: combining these would give a matrix of 32 (8×4) indices of health or health states (Table 7.2). Taking the scale from 1 to 0 meaning healthy to dead, any negative value denotes a state worse than death (e.g. confined to bed and in severe distress, cell D7 in the matrix). The matrix has recently been expanded into three dimensions.

Table 7.2 *The Rosser et al. matrix*

| | | Distress rating | | | |
		A	B	C	D
	Disability rating	None	Mild	Moderate	Severe
1	No disability	1.000	0.995	0.990	0.967
2	Slight social disability	0.990	0.986	0.973	0.932
3	Severe social disability	0.980	0.972	0.956	0.912
4	Work limited	0.964	0.956	0.942	0.870
5	Unable to work	0.946	0.935	0.900	0.700
6	Confined to chair	0.875	0.845	0.680	0.000
7	Confined to bed	0.677	0.564	0.000	−1.486
8	Unconscious	−1.0028	na	na	na

These valuations were derived from a sample of 70 people which included patients, doctors, nurses, and healthy volunteers.
na, not applicable.

The Rosser *et al.* matrix has provoked various points of debate. Two of the health states in the matrix had negative numerics and since death had the numeric of zero this suggested that there were conditions worse than death. One interpretation of health gain here is that people who fall into the two negative states would be better off dead. For those unconscious with no disability the health gain of dying would be 0−(−1.028) = 1.028. For those confined to bed with severe distress the health gain of dying would be 0–(–1.486) = 1.486. To make matters more complex, there is a suggestion in the matrix that a combined state of being confined to a chair and suffering severe distress is numerically the same as death. Such findings have naturally raised manifold problems and serious debate not least along ethical, planning, and resource decision making lines.

Cost measurers

Two areas need careful handling in value-for-money studies: first the nature of costs, and second how to find out how sensitive the results of analysis are to changes in the underlying factors. Table 7.3 identifies the various types of costs.

Table 7.3   *Types of cost*

Type of cost	Meaning
Sunk costs	Costs that are not recoverable
Fixed costs	Costs that are incurred regardless of number of clients treated
Variable costs	Costs that vary with the volume of patients
Total costs	Entire costs of the healthcare intervention
Average costs	Total costs divided by the quantity involved
Marginal costs	Incremental increase in total costs resulting from an incremental increase in quantity involved
Opportunity cost	Value of benefits foregone in programme A if programme B is chosen

Sunk costs are costs incurred in practice which are irretrievable. For, example a GP practice may buy some dedicated and specific clinical test equipment: that equipment cannot be used for anything except clinical testing. If that equipment has no other purpose and cannot easily be resold to another organization, then it represents a sunk cost for the practice. If a community trust spends money in advertising and promoting its services, then the costs incurred are sunk as once incurred they are irretrievable.

Fixed costs in healthcare are the overheads in hospitals and outreach clinics such as lighting, security, heating, general cleaning. Fixed costs do not vary with the level of activity.

An example of variable costs would be the costs of drugs. At one extreme if there are no patients on medication there are no drugs used so the variable cost would be zero but then the drugs bill increases the greater the number of patients who receive drugs. Variable costs are those costs that vary with the level of activity.

The total costs of healthcare intervention are composed of the fixed costs plus the variable costs. Total costs are not generally confined to the amount on the drugs bill for the fundholder or the health commission. The total costs of health-care intervention include the complete set of costs incurred by all parties in iden-tifying, processing, and caring for the patient. Thus the total cost will include costs incurred by the GP's time, the GP support staff time and administration expense, any hospital costs incurred (e.g. in clinical screening and laboratory testing of samples), any district nursing costs incurred, and the patient's costs incurred in getting to the clinics. If the patient is subsequently cared for in a local authority home then that cost can be considered part of the total cost of the healthcare intervention.

The calculation of marginal costs involves determining the incremental increase in total costs resulting from an incremental increase in quantity involved. Therefore marginal costs (and calculations of marginal benefits) helps to establish how much of a good or service to use rather than whether or not to use it at all. This is important when deciding to change the intensity of use of goods or services, rather than whether to use them at all.

In deciding on the course of care for the patient, healthcare professionals often face more than one choice. We noted above the choice between pro-gramme A or programme B in the treatment of ventricular arrhythmias. If the choice is to go for programme A rather than programme B the value of benefits that could have come from programme B represent the 'opportunity cost' of choosing programme A.

The results of economic analysis will therefore depend on the types of costs considered. Table 7.4 indicates the nature of costs and benefits (outcomes) of healthcare intervention: direct costs and benefits; indirect costs and benefits; and intangible costs and benefits.

Table 7.4 *The nature of costs and benefits*

Costs	Examples	Benefits (outcomes)
Direct	Clinic administration	Clinical, psychological
Indirect	Costs incurred by patients	Patient gets back to work
Intangible	Pain, anxiety, distress	Spiritual and emotional gains from relief from sickness

Sensitivity analysis

All value-for-money studies have certain assumptions or parameters underlying their results, so it is useful to see how the results of the study change as the under-lying factors are changed. In addition to a theoretical interest, are there any prac-tical reasons for determining the response of the results of value-for-money studies to changes in the underlying parameters? In fact, there are various practical reasons for using sensitivity analysis. For example, how would the results change:

- if there was an increase or reduction in the number of patients accessing the service
- if the costs of care differed over time or between locations in the country
- if primary care professionals introduced better patient selection systems, which in turn may result in fewer but higher cost patients being cared for.

Practical reasons also exist where we are genuinely uncertain about the volumes or costs involved.

When purchasing, providing or reading an economic assessment of healthcare intervention, it is important to appreciate the various types of errors that can be encountered in economic analysis. Box 7.1 summarizes the 10 most common mistakes.

Box 7.1 *The 10 most common mistakes in economic assessment*

1. Asking the wrong question
2. Not answering the question set
3. Using the wrong method of analysis
4. Not capturing costs appropriately
5. Not measuring benefits appropriately
6. Ignoring non-health sector costs and benefits
7. Not performing a sensitivity analysis
8. Study conclusions not derived from study results
9. Not identifying the alternative treatment paths completely
10. Not making explicit the sponsors of the study

It should not be thought that economic assessment of healthcare intervention abrogates primary healthcare professionals' autonomy or clinical freedom. That is not the purpose of health economics: its purpose is to offer a framework for making more explicit the resource implications, costs, and benefits of decisions or actions. In doing so it helps identify where room for improvement in decision making exists. Health economics provides information to decision makers and stakeholders: it does not provide decision makers any escape from making decisions.

Further reading

Andres, E., Temme, M., Radershatt, B., Szecsenyi, J., Sandholzer, H., Kochen, M. M. (1995). COOP-WONCA charts: a suitable functional status screening instrument in acute low back pain? *British Journal of General Practice*, **45**, 661–4.

Barber, N. (1995). What constitutes good prescribing? *British Medical Journal*, **310**, 923–5.

Bowling, A. (1997). *Measuring health: a review of quality of life measurement scales*, 2nd edn. Open University Press, Buckingham.

Canadian Coordinating Office for Health Technology Assessment (1994). *Guidelines for economic evaluation of medicines*. CCOHTA, Ottawa, Canada.

Commonwealth of Australia (1995). *Guidelines for the pharmaceutical industry on the preparation of submissions to the Pharmaceutical Benefits Advisory Committee: Including submissions involving economic analysis.* Department of Health, Housing and Community Services, Canberra, Australia.

Drummond, M., Maynard, A. (eds) (1993). *Purchasing and providing cost-effective health care.* Churchill Wheatsheaf, London.

Earl-Slater, A., Fitzmaurice, D., Wilcox, V. (1997). Assessing GP fundholding. *Primary Care Management*, **6**, 6–11.

Earl-Slater, A., Hobbs, R., Knight, J., Saviour, W. (1996). Evidence based prescribing in primary care. *Primary Care Management*, **6**, 6–10.

Earl-Slater, A. (1996). Setting priorities in the NHS. *British Journal of Health Care Management*, **2**, 19–23.

Fitzpatrick, R., Fletcher, A., Gore, S., Jones, D., Speighalter, D., Cox, D. (1992). Quality of life measures in health care: applications and issues in assessment. *British Medical Journal*, **305**, 1074–7.

Fletcher, A., Gore, S., Jones, D., Fitzpatrick, R., Speighalter, D., Cox, D. (1992). Quality of life measures in health care: design, analysis and interpretation. *British Medical Journal*, **305**, 1145–8.

Gillman, S. J., Ball, M., Prasad, M., Dunne, H., Cohen, S., Vafids, G. (1995). Investigation of the benefits and costs of an ophthalmic outreach clinic in general practice. *British Journal of General Practice*, **45**, 649–52.

Harris, C. (ed.) (1996). *Prescribing in general practice: the business side of general practice.* Radcliffe Medical Press, Oxford.

Hutchinson, A., McColl, E., Christie, M., Riccalton, C. (eds) (1996). *Health outcome measures in primary and out-patient care.* Harwood Academic, Amsterdam.

Jefferson, T., Demicheli, V., Mugford, M. (1996). *Elementary economic evaluation in health care.* BMJ Publishing, London.

Jenkinson, C. (ed.) (1994). *Measuring health and medical outcomes.* UCL Press, London.

Kinnersley, P., Peters, T., Stott, N. (1994). Measuring functional status in primary care. *British Journal of General Practice*, **44**, 545–51.

Langham, S., Thorogood, M., Normand, C., Muir, J., Jones, L., Fowler, G. (1996). Costs and cost effectiveness of health checks conducted by nurses in primary care: the Oxcheck study. *British Medical Journal*, **312**, 1265–8.

McAlister, D. (1990). Option appraisal: turning an Art into a Science? *Public Money and Management*, Winter, 43–50.

McKell, D., Stewart, A. (1994). A cost-minimisation analysis comparing topical versus systemic NSAIDs in the treatment of mild osteoarthritis of the superficial joints. *British Journal of Medical Economics*, **7**, 137–146.

Mooney, G. (1994). *Key issues in health economics.* Harvester Wheatsheaf, London.

Pickering, W. G. (1996). Does medical treatment mean patient benefit? *Lancet*, **347**, 370–80.

Revicki, D. A., Brown, R. E., Palmer, W., Bakish, D., Rosser, W. W., Anoton, S. F., Feeny, D. (1995). Modelling the cost effectiveness of antidepressant treatment in primary care. *Pharmacoeconomics*, **8**, 524–40.

Robinson, R. (1993). Economic evaluation and health care: What does it mean? *British Medical Journal*, **307**, 670–3.

Robinson, R. (1993). Economic evaluation and health care: costs and cost minimisation analysis. *British Medical Journal*, **307**, 726–8.

Robinson, R. (1993). Economic evaluation and health care: cost effectiveness analysis. *British Medical Journal*, **307**, 793–5.

Robinson, R. (1993). Economic evaluation and health care: cost utility analysis. *British Medical Journal*, **307**, 859–62.

Robinson, R. (1993). Economic evaluation and health care: cost benefit analysis. *British Medical Journal*, **307**, 924–6.

Robinson, R. (1993). Economic evaluation and health care: the policy context. *British Medical Journal*, **307**, 994–6.

Royal College of Physicians (1995). *Setting priorities in the NHS: a framework for decision making.* Royal College of Physicians, London.

Sloane, E. (ed.) (1996). *Valuing health care: costs benefits, and effectiveness of pharmaceuticals and other medical technologies.* Cambridge University Press, Cambridge.

Spiegelhalter, D. J., Gore, S. M., Fitzpatrick, R., Fletcher, A. E., Jones, D. R., Cox, D. R. (1992). Quality of life measures in health care: resource allocation. *British Medical Journal*, **305**, 1205–9.

Stewart, S., Glynn, J. G., Perkins, D. A. (1996). *Achieving value for money.* W. B. Saunders, London.

Streiner, D. L., Norman, G. (1995). *Health measurement scales: a practical guide*, 2nd edn. Oxford University Press, Oxford.

Szczepura, A., Kankaanpa, J. (eds) (1996). *Assessment of health care technologies: case studies, key concepts and strategic issues.* Wiley, New York.

Toon, P. (1994). *What is good general practice?* Royal College of General Practitioners, London.

CHAPTER EIGHT

Impact of the UK healthcare reforms on prescribing

Tom Walley, John Ferguson, and Yvonne Carter

Prescribing by GPs has come in for extensive attention in recent years, because of the rising costs, concerns about the quality of much prescribing, and value for money. This increased attention must, however, be seen in the context of extensive reforms in the NHS over the same period, the biggest upheaval since its inception in the 1940s.

The NHS reforms

The UK government undertook radical and controversial changes to the organisation and delivery of healthcare in the early 1990s, with the aim of improving services for patients, while making better use of resources and integrating care across the primary, secondary, and private sectors. Latterly, an important element of these reforms has been the explicit recognition of the great strengths of British primary care, and its cost effectiveness. Hence the reforms have refocused on encouraging the development of a primary care led NHS rather than a traditional hospital dominated NHS.

The NHS changes followed two broad and related themes. The first was the development of an internal NHS market whereby the health service may be broadly divided into purchasers of healthcare (e.g. health authorities or GP fundholders) and providers (e.g. self-governing trust hospitals or other NHS or private organizations), and assuming that competition between providers would lead to improvement in services. The second theme was the devolvement of responsibility for services away from central government and on to local bodies, either as purchasers or as providers.

Before 1990, primary care was undertaken by GPs working as independent contractors with a broad and poorly defined contract, and administered but not managed by the Family Practitioner Committee (FPC). As a first step in moving to a primary care led health service, the government decided that there was currently inadequate management of primary care and replaced the FPCs with Family Health Service Authorities (FHSAs), which were to actively manage primary care in their area. The power to do this came in part from the imposition, despite much hostility from the British Medical Association, of a new GP contract. This contract introduced an element of performance-related pay to GP reimbursement for the first time, dependent on achieving targets for vaccinations and other areas. It also made individual GPs more accountable to the FHSA for their hours of work and the type and quality of service. FHSAs were in turn answerable to the Regional Health Authority, which up to then had paid little attention to and had little understanding of primary care, and which was in many cases disconcerted by this new responsibility. (Although FHSAs have been replaced since 1996 by merged health authorities, as of 1997 PACT data still uses this term to designate local health authority comparison figures.)

In 1994, the reforms went further still. It became apparent that the divisions of healthcare into primary care (managed by the FHSA) and secondary care (managed by the District Health Authority), under the overall stewardship of the Regional Health Authority, were no longer appropriate, and were wasteful. The advent and expansion of GP fundholding, which spanned both primary and secondary care, highlighted this further. The government undertook to merge the District Health Authorities (DHAs) and FHSAs into one combined health commission, which would purchase services for its population, and would be directly answerable not to a Regional Health Authority (which would cease to exist), but to a local office of the NHS Executive. The merged authorities or commissions came into being in April 1996.

Prescribing and the NHS reforms

Running alongside these far-reaching reforms of the health service were a series of initiatives designed to address the on-going concern about the size of the nation's drugs bill. This increased on average at a rate of 4% above inflation over 1981–91 (Government Statistical Service, 1996). The Department of Health (DoH) considered that such rises, coupled with financial restrictions being placed on the health service as a whole, would lead to cuts elsewhere in the NHS. This led to further attempts to control drug expenditure, particularly in primary care where 80% of drug expenditure occurs. Furthermore, prescribing comprises about 50% of total primary care expenditure, and in the new managed NHS primary care, no manager could ignore such a large part of the budget. Such concerns about rising drug bills are not confined to the UK, but are common throughout the developed world.

There were grounds for the frequently stated anxiety that prescribing was sometimes unnecessary and wasteful. Considerable variations in the average per capita rates of prescribing and costs of drugs in different areas of the UK, and even between neighbouring practices, had been observed. Differences across the country are only partly explained by different age structures of the population in different areas, as well as poverty and morbidity (e.g. between affluent Oxford where prescribing cost £58.37 per head in 1994, and the more deprived Liverpool at £81.25 per head) (Prescription Pricing Authority, 1995). The variations in GPs' prescribing rates and costs can also be explained in some part on the same grounds, since particular practices may attract certain patients or types of patient, but the single greatest factor in this variation is the doctor (see further discussion in Chapter 2).

Apart from the financial concerns, such variability in prescribing practice supports concerns about the quality and appropriateness of prescribing in primary care—are some patients being overtreated unnecessarily, exposing them to risk and wasting resources, or are others being inadequately treated? Most likely, both are true in different settings. These financial and quality considerations lead to concerted government action around prescribing becoming inevitable. Their action was partly education based and partly managerial, and was set out in the DoH (1990) publication 'Improving Prescribing'.

The principle initiative described here is the Indicative Prescribing Scheme (IPS). Other elements were to include

- the appointment of medical and, possibly, pharmaceutical advisers to FHSAs
- the provision of more independent advice on drugs from the newly constituted Medicines Resource Centre in Liverpool
- the promotion of medical audit (particularly of prescribing) which was to be aided by the provision of PACT data (see below)
- the promotion of prescribing formularies and generic prescribing particularly
- more research into prescribing to be executed by the Prescribing Research Unit to be based at the University of Leeds.

Optional elements, to which GPs could subscribe on a voluntary basis, were the incentive schemes (see below) and the GP fundholding scheme (see below) which includes an allocation for drugs as a major component of the total budget. The reward for opting in was the possibility of retaining some or all of any savings on drug costs for redeployment into other areas of practice development. The initiatives were backed by the threat of sanctions if doctors were deemed to be prescribing excessively and a new mechanism for dealing with allegations of excessive prescribing was laid down. The net effects of various parts of these actions are often difficult to disentangle.

The Indicative Prescribing Scheme

The IPS scheme was developed by the DoH with the initial aim of

placing downward pressure on expenditure on drugs, particularly in those practices with the highest expenditure, but without in any way preventing people getting the medicines they need (DoH, 1990).

This emphasis on costs provoked considerable hostility and, when it finally appeared, the emphasis changed to improving the quality of prescribing and cost effectiveness, with cost savings as a secondary benefit.

From April 1991, GPs were set an indicative prescribing amount (IPA), intended to cover the costs of their prescribing for the following year. The IPA was based on the previous year's spending, modified by an 'uplift' factor determined by central government, and adjusted locally to meet special needs by a medical or pharmacist prescribing adviser to the local FHSA (see below). Practitioners then receive monthly statements showing their actual spend compared to their predicted spend; in theory, if they find themselves overspending, GPs might modify their future prescribing to keep within their overall IPA. Likewise, if the FHSA prescribing adviser detected a developing overspend in a practice, this would be an indication for a visit to discuss prescribing issues, at which the practice might be asked to justify any overspend on clinical grounds.

The prescribing adviser would take the opportunity of setting the IPA to engage the practice in discussions around prescribing including such factors as perceived over- or underprescribing, and specific clinical aspects. The practice is supposed to agree the IPA, as an amount within which they will endeavour to keep their prescribing costs.

In practice, the scheme has suffered from many problems. These included

- the use of historic prescribing costs to calculate the future amount, so penalizing previously careful prescribers and rewarding the higher cost or volume prescribers
- unrealistic uplift factors below the rate of inflation, which resulted in low amounts which were impossible to implement
- the lack of real penalties for 'overspending' practitioners (although penalties do exist for extreme cases of overprescribing, they are difficult to apply)
- the lack of incentives to encourage 'savings'
- the general antagonism of GPs for any government attempt to curb costs, in part fuelled by poor understanding of the complex scheme.

Furthermore, since the IPA represents only a theoretical budget, not a real one, savings or overspends are also theoretical.

Even within health authorities, there was confusion about what the IPA represented: a projected out-turn on the year's spending, a target to be aimed for, the maximum permissible spend, or just an administrative measure of no real significance? It is hardly surprising, therefore, that GPs often simply ignored the IPA. As a result, in 1991–92, 85% of GP practices 'overspent' their IPA, while in 1992–93, the total 'overspend' among non fundholding practices was 7.5% of the predicted budget; and the scheme 'has been somewhat discredited to date as a means of controlling expenditure' (Audit Commission, 1994).

However, the IPS was only part of a broader initiative to improve prescribing, some parts of which have been successful. Prescribing advisers have volunteered examples of improved quality of prescribing in individual practices as a result of their interventions, or can point to a rise in the rate of generic prescribing. But quality of prescribing is not often quantifiable and certainly not highly visible, unlike cost.

Since no formal evaluation has been conducted, it is unclear to what extent the drug bill might have risen in the absence of the IPS. The IPS was introduced at a time when the drug bill was undergoing an almost unprecedented rise. The DoH suggests that the single biggest factor in the rising drug bill is a change in product mix, with new more expensive drugs, replacing older and less expensive drugs. It is certainly possible that the IPS has had some effect in containing the impact of such new products on the drugs bill. There are also year-on-year modifications to the scheme to try and address some of the criticisms. Thus changes are now being made to the budget setting process to move away from historic spend baselines and to base budgets on a form of weighted capitation which it is hoped will reflect more closely actual need from medicines.

In conjuction with the budget setting process and financial pressures applied to GPs regarding their prescribing, the IPS has also aspired to rely on an educational approach at least running in parallel.

Prescribing information and education initiatives

Information and education initiatives aim to promote GP awareness of the costs, rates, and details of their prescribing, and seemed in a pilot trial to encourage more rational and cost-effective prescribing (Harris *et al.*, 1984). Specifically, they include

- the provision of data to GPs on all drugs issued on their prescription with emphasis on cost (PACT data, see below)
- the provision of drug information to GPs by bulletins, including a new one to be produced by the Medicines Resource Centre mentioned above
- the activities of professional medical or pharmaceutical advisers, including the promotion of generic prescribing and the use of formularies.

Prescribing Analysis and CosT (PACT)

From the early days of the NHS, data had been gather on the costs associated with prescribing of individual doctors. This formed the basis of a scheme whereby doctors whose prescribing costs were seen to deviate significantly from that or their peers would be visited by the Regional Medical Officer. With the computerization of the Prescription Pricing Authority (PPA) it became possible to speed up and develop this system.

The first computerized information system was based on the preceding manual PD2/PD8 system. Experience with this system led to the development of a more informative and selective information system named PACT (Prescribing Analysis and CosT). To ensure that the PACT system met the needs of GPs, a user group with members from the DoH, Prescription Pricing Authority, General Medical Services Committee, Royal College of GPs, Royal Pharmaceutical Society, and Society of FPS Administrators was set up. It was decided to produce a system which would provide GPs with well-presented, timely, and frequent information. In order to ensure that users were not swamped with information, the system was designed to present the information at three different levels, depending on the needs of the GP.

This PACT system was implemented in August 1988. Every month approximately 8000 GPs received a summary of their prescribing for the previous quarter in the form of an automatic level I report. Level II reports highlighted the areas of prescribing where the major costs were incurred and were 'remedial' in the sense that they were sent automatically to GPs whose overall prescribing costs had exceeded a predetermined threshold. Level III reports were only issued at the request of individual practitioners, as they contained a full catalogue of all the prescriptions issued during the quarter and provided a level of detail which was only useful to those interested in self-audit of their prescribing or in the development of formularies or practice protocols.

The Leeds PACT pilot scheme demonstrated that substantial savings in the drug budget can be achieved using PACT, through generic prescribing, therapeutic substitution, and reducing inappropriate prescribing. Spencer and van Zwanenberg (1989) reported that PACT was a vast improvement over the PD8 scheme, especially in the presentation of data, but that it had limitations as it did not identify clinical factors or repeat prescribing. Within a year of the introduction of PACT and the receipt by GPs of details of their prescribing, the PPA was able to show that the number of high-spending doctors was decreasing, suggesting that feedback works.

In 1991 the NHS Management Executive called for a more integrated approach to the planning, management and delivery of primary and secondary healthcare including pharmaceutical services, and stated that the rational effective use of medicines requires pharmacists to work in close collaboration with doctors, nurses and other health and social care professions.

As a result of these changes and in response to criticisms of the existing system it was decided that the PACT reports should be updated and improved. Extensive consultation was undertaken with the profession and all those interested in prescribing information and, wherever possible, their suggestions were incorporated into the new PACT reports (Anon, 1994). These were designed to be high quality, user-friendly reports with additional features such as the practice's top 20 drugs and the proportion of new drugs included for the first time. These standard PACT reports replace the previous level I and II reports and, within a standard format, they contain much practice-specific prescribing information. These reports are sent to all GPs in England every 3 months towards the end of February, May, August, and November. The previous streaming of reports has been discontinued so that these reports are now all directly comparable, with the PPA producing some 29 000 individual prescribing reports from its mainframe information computer through a high speed laser printer in the course of some 10 working days.

The important features of these new reports are highlighted in Table 8.1, along with suggestions as to how the information can be used to monitor prescribing.

Table 8.1 *Details of the PACT standard report* (see Appendix III, page 201, for example)

The PACT standard report
Page 1

Page 1 shows a simple bar chart of the practice's prescribing costs for the quarter compared with the FHSA equivalent (average) and the national equivalent (average). The FHSA equivalent is based on the actual figures for the local FHSA adjusted to create an imaginary practice with the same make-up of patients and age ranges. The national equivalent is created in the same way. These equivalents allow practices to see how their prescribing compares with other practices in the FHSA or nationally. The individual GP's prescribing costs are also shown. Figures are also given to show how these various costs have changed from the previous year.

Page 2

On page 2 the practice prescribing costs (and FHSA equivalents) are broken down into the national top 6 BNF therapeutic areas, currently (in order) gastro-intestinal, cardiovascular, respiratory, central nervous system, endocrine,   musculoskeletal and joint disease, and other. Alongside the costs in each therapeutic area, for the first time, is a figure giving the percentage of the prescribing costs in each area that are due to new drugs. Drugs are defined as 'new' for 3 years after their introduction (only new drugs that carry the CSM's black triangle symbol are included).

Also on this page is a list of the 20 leading-cost drugs in the practice giving the number of prescriptions, their total cost, the percentage of the practice total and the change from last year. In addition, brand-name drugs in the list are flagged with a 'G' if a generic preparation is available.

Page 3

This page concentrates on the number of items prescribed rather than costs. An item is equivalent to each order for a product written on an FP10, but the size of an item (amount prescribed) is not considered. For example, a prescription for 10 paracetamol tablets is considered as one item, as is a prescription for 100 paracetamol tablets. The chart shows:
- the number of items prescribed by the practice compared with FHSA and national equivalents
- the percentage of items written generically
- the percentage actually dispensed generically.

These figures are different because prescriptions may be written generically for products that are not available as a generic preparation and therefore the brand is dispensed. The number of items prescribed is then broken down into the various therapeutic areas.

Page 4

Page 4 combines the elements of the earlier data to provide details of the average cost per item for the practice compared to the FHSA and national equivalents.

The average costs per item are also shown in each of the therapeutic areas. The average cost per item will depend largely on the amount prescribed on each prescription and may reflect practice policy. If costs per item vary widely from the averages this may stimulate the practice to explore why.

Page 5

Six line graphs on page 5 show the changes in practice prescribing costs and FHSA equivalents over the last eight quarters in the six therapeutic areas, showing:

- how prescribing policy changes affect costs, e.g. increased use of anti-inflammatories in asthma
- whether the practice spending is converging or diverging from local patterns of prescribing.

Pages 6 and 7

An extensive table on pages 6 and 7 ranks the practice's own top 40 sections of the BNF in terms of cost. The number of items prescribed in each section is given along with comparisons with the FHSA and the practice's last year figures. This table allows the practice to identify the therapeutic sections that account for the largest proportion of its spending on drugs. These might be the sections that the practice may wish to concentrate its attention on through the use of the more detailed information available in the Prescribing Catalogue (see below).

Page 8

Practice details such as list size are carried on the back page together with details of items personally administered or dispensed by the practice. These items are those which attract payment under paragraph 44.5 of the Statement of Fees and Allowances (Red Book). A glossary of terms is also included on this page.

Centre pages

There is an insert in the centre of the standard PACT report detailing important and topical aspects of prescribing in general practice. It is illustrated by national trends in prescribing for this clinical indication, concentrating upon quality issues. There is additional practice-specific prescribing feedback related to the topic of the centre pages. The editor of this section is the Medical Director of the PPA and there is a multidisciplinary editorial board.

The Prescribing Catalogue

Prescribing Catalogues are available only on request. The report provides details of every item prescribed and dispensed by the practice or individual doctor, and the full report runs to about 100 pages. A Prescribing Catalogue can be requested for the practice overall or for individual partners or trainees. To avoid being overwhelmed by paper, doctors can request Prescribing Catalogues for six individual therapeutic areas.

The first few pages of the report repeat information provided in the Standard

Report and give additional details of prescribing rates. The remainder sets out in detail every item that has been dispensed in the quarter, with the quantity prescribed and total cost. The Catalogue also flags products available generically (GFA), new drugs (N), controlled drugs (CD), CSM monitored drugs (CSM), and borderline substances (BS).

The Prescribing Catalogue is by far the more valuable of the two reports if a practice wants to look in detail at its prescribing patterns and wants to monitor the effects of any changes in prescribing policy. The sheer volume of information provided in the reports can be daunting, but the key to success is to tackle it in manageable pieces.

Limitations and pitfalls of PACT

PACT data are extremely valuable but, as with any statistical information, they have their limitations and potential pitfalls. GPs need to be aware of these in order to avoid drawing the wrong conclusions and using the data inappropriately.

Comparisons with FHSA and national equivalents

The population characteristics of an individual practice are unique and can vary enormously from health authority and national equivalents. Prescribing in any practice is determined in part by the characteristics of the patient population. When comparing prescribing with local and national averages certain factors need to be borne in mind, as PACT data will not usually take account of them.

Prescribing units

PACT data recognize that elderly patients generally require more prescriptions than other age groups. Thus for comparative purposes the patient population is described by prescribing units (PUs). Under this system each patient over 65 is designated as counting for 3 PUs on the crude basis that these patients require on average three times as many prescriptions as under 65s.

The bar charts in the Standard PACT Report compare individual practices with a fictional 'average' or equivalent practice. The figures for this average practice are obtained by dividing the total costs or total number of prescriptions in the health authority in that quarter by the total number of PUs in the health authority. This give an average cost or number of prescriptions per PU in the health authority. These figures are then multiplied by the number of PUs in individual practices to give the costs and number of prescriptions for a practice of similar size and age profile prescribing at the average rate for the health authority.

ASTRO PUs

The Prescribing Research Unit in Leeds has developed a formula, the Age, Sex and Temporary Resident Prescribing Unit (ASTRO PU), that takes greater account of the differing prescribing needs of males and females in nine different age bands. This new formula allows more accurate comparisons between practices and is now used to help calculate prescribing budgets (Roberts and Harris, 1993).

Practice list size

The prescribing and cost rates given in PACT are based on the practice list size held by the health authority. Although this is appropriate in areas where the population is stable, prescribing and cost rates may not be accurate where the list size is rapidly changing. Data for individual partners are also based on their personal list size, so unless GPs only see patients registered with them, individual comparisons with practice and other equivalents are of little value (Harris *et al.*, 1990).

Cost per item

When looking at cost per item for the practice compared with health authority and national averages it is important to remember that this figure depends on the quantity of drug prescribed each time. A practice that always prescribes repeat prescriptions for 3 months will have a higher cost per item than a practice that prescribes 1 month's treatment. Cost per item should be looked at in conjunction with the number of items prescribed.

Practice or doctor data

PACT data for individual practitioners relate to the prescriptions written on that doctor's prescription pad or under that doctor's unique prescriber number. Where one doctor's FP10s are used for repeats or nurse-requested items, or where the trainee uses the trainer's pad, the PACT data can be distorted. For audit purposes aggregated practice data should be requested.

Medical and pharmaceutical advisers to health authorities

The DoH proposed that FHSAs should use independent medical advisers who would

encourage good practice in the referral of patients to hospital; be given a role in encouraging effective and economic prescribing and advise the Authority regarding its more active role in promoting service developments (DoH, 1990).

Medical advisers were appointed when the Local Medical Committee (LMC)-nominated GP members of what were then FPCs ceased to be an appropriate source of advice after the contract changed in 1990. Since then general medical and prescribing advice has been provided, independent of the LMC (the body representing and composed of GPs), by a medical prescribing adviser. This was a doctor experienced in general practice who would command the respect and co-operation of local GPs, and who would act as an adviser on the one hand to the FHSA and on the other to the GPs on prescribing issues.

Those taking up these posts who had made a career change to full-time medical advising had a variety of motivations: some were 'elder statesmen' who saw the post as a useful way to spend their time up to retirement; others were 'young Turks' who had visions of a primary care led NHS and wished to be part of the leadership (Walley and Bligh, 1992). Some were, in the words of one adviser, 'refugees from the new contract' who felt it was easier to apply the contract to their colleagues than to work under it. Many FHSAs appointed part-time medical advisers.

Although appointed to monitor prescribing issues, many medical advisers, as the sole professional adviser within the FHSA, found themselves taking on other duties around the management of primary care, not originally part of their remit, and leaving little time for prescribing. To address perceived learning needs, the National Medical Advisers' Support Centre (MASC) offered a wide spectrum of courses including negotiating skills, health economics, prescribing, and management. Health authorities increasingly also employed pharmacists to support prescribing matters, and in some authorities medical advisers have little or no role in prescribing.

Many medical advisers and pharmaceutical advisers were not appointed until shortly before the IPS came into operation. These resulted in the time available for consultation and discussion on IPAs at the practice level being much less than that desired by either side in the first year, with subsequent misunderstanding on both sides about intention and motivation. Many medical advisers were distrusted by their former colleagues, and faced some antagonism and hostility in their attempts to discuss prescribing. As time has gone on, the role of the medical adviser as a bridge between the health authority and the GP has become established with general acceptance by GPs.

Prescribing role of professional advisers

Professional advisers have come to fulfill the following major roles with regard to prescribing:

- Performing individual practice visits: to compare practice prescribing with health authority average; discussion of treatment consensus among partners; prescribing expenditure in relation to practice IPA; prescribing component of fundholding budgets; the need for repeat prescribing systems; to identify priority training areas and how they can be met.
- Assisting GPs to determine their requirements for prescribing at the primary–secondary care interface and ensure that purchasers include these criteria in contracts, such as the development of drug treatment protocols, specific policies on the use of drugs, shared care protocols for new drugs, and practice or district formularies.
- Ensuring that primary care concerns are heard and addressed at drug and therapeutics committees.
- Providing prescribing information for GPs in a relevant form, e.g. newsletter, information sheets, educational meetings.

- Developing areas of research and audit with GPs evaluating, for example, how consultation and prescribing rates relate to measures of deprivation and practice population characteristics; or the developing role of community pharmacists in improved prescribing.

However, the role of the primary care medical adviser has dwindled within the health authority with the merger of the DHA and FHSA. DHAs generally had the stronger management structures. This has led to some public health doctors, usually with little understanding or experience of primary care, attempting to act as directors of primary care, and displacing medical advisers with their GP background. However, it is clear that to function adequately in the new authorities, medical advisers will need to take on some of the skills of the public health doctor, including research skills, and that training as a GP alone will not suffice.

The medical adviser to a health commission should play a key role in developing relationships with GPs across a range of primary/community healthcare management and health commissioning issues. Primary responsibilities will be to develop policy for primary care, lead on prescribing, and advise on primary care development and its links with secondary care commissioning. In some areas the adviser will be a senior member of the senior management team for a commission.

Pharmaceutical advisers, although orginally suggested only as an optional source of prescribing advice, have been more successful in establishing their role, because of their narrower and clearer remit within health authorities. Initially they frequently had difficulties in discussing prescribing with GPs, because of their relative lack of understanding of primary care, and because of their inexperience at directly prescribing themselves. This diminished their credibility with GPs, who nevertheless often saw them as less threatening than, and hence preferable to, medical advisers. As they have gained experience, they have overcome many of these difficulties and often taken on almost sole responsibility for prescribing matters within the health authority.

The GP fundholding scheme

Under the GP fundholding scheme, as originally constructed, large practices could hold a budget for spending on behalf of their patients on all non-acute hospital therapeutic and diagnostic services, any drugs prescribed or dispensed, as well as all practice expenses. Spending in fundholding practices is monitored by the health authority, to detect overspends and maintain clinical standards if necessary. The scheme is structured so that doctors should not have personal financial incentives, but so that practices are able to improve their services for the benefit of patients, by moving money within their overall budget between different aspects of that service. This, and the ability to force local providers to be more responsive to the demands of the practice, have been the main attractions of the scheme.

Like many of the reforms, this scheme divided the profession. After an initially slow take-up, numbers of applications have grown. The entry criteria have also become less stringent so as to encourage smaller practices or even single handed practices (linked in consortia). By April 1996, 50% of all GPs were fundholders.

Fundholding fitted with the political philosophy of the government, and this political imperative hampered attempts to evaluate its success. Administrative costs of the NHS have increased drastically, partly as a result of fundholding by as much as £100 million per annum. The political aspects of fundholding have resulted in its future remaining uncertain. Even within practices, fundholding also seems unstable. In surveys of fundholding GPs, only two thirds of responders said that they supported the scheme; many GPs are keen on the responsiveness to local demands which fundholding has brought, but would be happy with alternative models of purchasing which are being explored in some areas, such as GP consortia or locality purchasing.

A development of fundholding is total GP purchasing, whereby fundholders hold budgets for all services for their patients, and not just the limited budgets currently held. This is currently (1996) being piloted.

Prescribing by GP fundholders

GP fundholders have a clear incentive to restrain cost rises in their drug bill, which is in practice the component of the budget where it is most possible to make savings. Although savings made were to be used for patient benefits, there had been concern that some fundholders may have benefited, with first wave fundholders on average keeping £50 000 of their allocated budget. Early anomalies in the scheme which may have led to overfunding (including loose budget setting because of lack of accurate information particularly about hospital referral rates and costs), have now been largely eliminated.

Studies of prescribing in fundholders have mostly looked at small numbers of first wave fundholders, who were not typical GPs (Bradlow and Coulter, 1993; Maxwell et al., 1993; Glennester et al., 1994). Fundholders have contained the rise in the drug bill more effectively than non-fundholders; in 1992–93 net ingredient costs rose by 10–13% for fundholders and by 19% for non-fundholders (Bradlow and Coulter, 1993). Many fundholding practices made a saving on their drug budget, while non-fundholders exceeded their IPAs. However, these figures are not strictly comparable since some of the fundholders were given a slightly more generous budget than justified by their historical spending, as part of a policy of the Regional Health Authorities.

A report by the Audit Commission in 1992/3 looked at prescribing by a large number of fundholding practices (249, out of a total of approximately 1400 fundholding practices at the time) and non-fundholding practices (3120 out of a total of approximately 9800). They showed that fundholders prescribed at lower cost per prescribing unit by an average of 9.4%, and that the rate of increase of prescribing costs in fundholders (10% in first wave fundholders but only 7.7% in second wave) was less than in non-fundholders (12%); nationally, the rate of rise of costs in fundholders was 4% lower than in non-fundholders. Fundholders also prescribed more generic preparations and spent about a quarter less on drugs of limited or no clinical value, and on antibiotics. As a marker of quality of prescribing, fundholders prescribed 0.33 DDDs of inhaled corticosteroids per DDD of inhaled bronchodilator, compared to 0.3 for non-fundholders, suggesting that the patients of fundholders were not being deprived of necessary treatment in areas of evident medical need.

In general, therefore, early wave fundholders reduced prescribing costs, or contained their rise, allowing them to make savings on their budget. They achieved these savings in part by eliminating unnecessary prescribing, by minimizing cost (by moving to generic prescribing); by altering their choice of drug within a therapeutic class on cost grounds (e.g. cimetidine for ranitidine); and, to a lesser extent, by reducing the volume of prescribing or containing its rise.

Early wave fundholders were largely well-organized and highly motivated enthusiasts for the government's reforms, and were drawn from more affluent areas. As such, they may have been traditionally low prescribers. Later waves have often included practices with no great interest in fundholding philosophically and who may even consider it unjust, but who nevertheless have become fundholders so as not to be left behind. The effectiveness of such practices in containing drug costs may therefore be less than that of the early wave fundholders (Stewart-Brown et al., 1995).

Prescribing incentive schemes

Incentive schemes were established to give non-fundholding GPs a direct incentive to save money on their IPA. Prescribing targets, which would save money and improve quality of prescribing, were set by agreement between the Local Medical Committee representing the GPs and the FHSA. If the target savings were achieved, half the savings generated were made available for agreed local projects for improving patient care. In the early years at least, these schemes were not popular and were generally unsuccessful.

However, the schemes have been resurrected with targets set 1–3% below the practice target budget—the exact target will be more 'challenging' for high prescribing practices. If a practice achieved this target or better, they may keep up to 35% of all savings (the exact amount is at the discretion of the FHSA prescribing adviser), to a maximum of £3000 per GP, to be used for patients' benefit. The targets may not be purely financial, but may include such things as a level of generic prescribing, use of a formulary, or control of repeat prescribing. Local variations in this scheme are allowed.

No details are available yet of the results of such schemes nationally, although it was rumoured that in the first year of the new incentive scheme, payments (about £7 million) were double what the DoH had anticipated, suggesting that the scheme was more successful than expected. Anecdotal reports from individual FHSAs support this. In 1995, the terms of such schemes were altered so that there was no formal admission to the scheme and any GP saving money on his or her prescribing budget and meeting other targets was entitled to payments. The funding for these extended incentive payments came largely from fundholding prescribing budgets, which were effectively reduced. Whether this reduced the incentive for fundholders to control their prescribing has not yet been studied.

Prescribing at the interface between primary and secondary care

Prescribing in hospitals has a major influence on prescribing in the community, and closer regulation of hospital prescribing could pay dividends in the community, particularly around choice of drug. Hospitals with responsibility only for their own drug budgets were happy to accept cut price deals on drugs from pharmaceutical companies, who in turn made large profits from community sales.

A further factor has been the cash-limited nature of hospital drug budgets, resulting in the 'cost shifting' of prescribing or expensive drugs such as erythropoietin or human growth hormone on to GPs, so that the total cost falls to their budget. This separation of prescribing from clinical responsibility (the GP who signs the prescription has legal responsibility for it, even though he has little true clinical responsibility) and from resources responsibility is unsatisfactory. Guidelines about both medical and financial responsibility for such treatments have been produced by the DoH, although there is still a major role for local agreements between hospital doctors and GPs. Purchasers, both health authorities and GP fundholders, now often include prescribing issues in their contracts with hospitals, including a requirement for the hospital to consider the costs of drugs in the community and not just in hospital when making formulary decisions.

Under the latest reforms, commissioning authorities have been created covering primary and secondary care. This may unify drug budgets across primary and secondary care and resolve the cost shifting and problems with clinical responsibility which this created. Combined primary and secondary care therapeutics committees are being established in many areas. Furthermore, purchasers are instructed by government to purchase services of proven efficacy, and this will inevitably start to restrain clinical freedom whereby each doctor treats patients as he sees fit, leading to variable quality of practice and inefficiency. Purchasers are likely therefore to seek to actively influence choice of drug and even the decision to prescribe in hospitals. In this they may be guided by the results of systematic reviews of the evidence of effectiveness, produced for instance by the Cochrane Centre, and also by economic evaluations of the cost effectiveness of therapies (see Chapters 6 and 7).

Conclusions

Prescribing in primary care is complex and expensive. The needs of consumers, prescribers, manufacturers, and government interact to make formal control over costs difficult. The most successful method of control so far has been to devolve direct responsibility for their drug spending to the prescribers, and include financial incentives. However, this might carry risks of harming patients unless quality of prescribing remains clearly on the government and professional agenda. There is a serious danger that consideration of cost may distract from consideration of quality. Ways of defining and measuring quality in prescribing need to be developed and reporting of such quality indicators provided to prescribers alongside cost data.

The problems around prescribing and its quality and cost have not been created by the NHS reforms. These problems are present world-wide, but the reforms have brought the issue to the fore as a major focus of GP activity. Difficulties around prescribing illustrate the difficulties which face UK healthcare, with demand and technical ability exceeding the resources to deliver them, while the government largely avoids issues of rationing of healthcare for fear of electoral disaster. These problems must be resolved in healthcare as a whole and not just in relation to prescribing.

There are many ambivalent attitudes in all players in prescribing:

- government wishes to contain the drug bill while supporting a powerful pharmaceutical industry
- prescribers wish to treat the patient and retain professional freedom and privilege, but recognize that they are perhaps failing at times to deliver value for money
- the public wants treatment, and new innovative medicines, while at the same time being probably reluctant to pay for such benefits either directly or in taxation.

These tensions underlie the relative failure of the IPS to control cost rises. Adding direct incentives to doctors to modify their prescribing, coupled with more realistic and accurate setting of budgets are an improvement. Whether such improvements are a prelude to the introduction of firm practice prescribing budgets for all GPs remains to be seen.

The possibilities for moving from consideration of drug costs to drug value and value for money seem limited at present, but the purchaser/provider split may offer some hope for the future.

References

Anon, (1994). *New PACT for GPs.* HMSO, London.

Audit Commission (1994). *A prescription for improvement—towards more rational prescribing in general practice.* Audit Commission, London.

Bradlow, J., Coulter, A. (1993). Effects of fundholding and indicative prescribing schemes on general practitioners' prescribing costs. *British Medical Journal*, **307**, 1186–9.

Department of Health (1990). *Improving prescribing*. HMSO, London.

Glennester, H., Matsanganis, M., Owen, P., Hancock, S. (1994). GP fundholding: wild-card or winning hand? In *Evaluating the NHS reforms*, ed. R. Robinson, J. LeGrand. King's Fund, London.

Government Statistical Service (1996). *Statistics of prescriptions dispensed in the Family Health Services Authorities: England 1985 to 1995*. HMSO, London.

Harris, C. M., Jarman, B., Woodman, E., White, P., Fry, J. (1984). *Prescribing—a suitable case for treatment*. Occasional Paper 24, Royal College of General Practitioners, Exeter.

Harris, C. M., Heywood, P. L., Clayden, A. D. (19??). *The analysis of prescribing in general practice—a guide to audit and research*. HMSO, London.

Maxwell, M., Heaney, D., Howie, J. G. R., Noble, S. (1993). General practice fundholding: observations on prescribing patterns and costs using the defined daily dose method. *British Medical Journal*, **307**, 1190–4.

Prescription Pricing Authority (1995). *Annual report*. Prescription Pricing Authority, Newcastle.

Roberts, S. J., Harris, C. M., (1993). Age, sex and temporary resident originated prescribing units (ASTRO-PUs) new weightings for analysing prescribing of general practice in England. *British Medical Journal*, **307**, 485–8.

Spencer, J. A., van Zwanenberg, T. D. (1991). Prescribing research: PACT to the future. *Journal of the Royal College of General Practitioners*, **39**, 270–2.

Stewart-Brown, S., Surender, R., Bradlow, J., Coulter, A., Doll, H. (1995). The effects of fundholding in general practice on prescribing habits three years after introduction of the scheme. *British Medical Journal*, **311**, 1543–7.

Walley, T., Bligh, J. (1992). FHSA medical advisers: friends or foes? *British Medical Journal*, **304**, 133–4.

CHAPTER NINE

Responding to changing healthcare systems: adapting prescribing in the new NHS

Colin Bradley and Alison Blenkinsopp

Given that the NHS reforms detailed in the preceding chapter have been implemented and are unlikely to be reversed by any subsequent administration, it is imperative that GPs adapt their practices to take account of these changed circumstances. It is no longer possible for GPs to prescribe for patients as they see fit without regard to the economic consequences of their actions. A major thrust of the new environment created by the reforms is to make doctors bear some financial, as well as clinical, responsibility for their prescribing.

This has several immediately obvious consequences for GPs. First, they must become more aware of the costs of the drugs they prescribe and, particularly, the cost differentials between alternative drug choices for the conditions they commonly treat. Second, when challenged about the costs of their prescribing, as within the new system GPs are bound to be, they can respond in one of two ways:

• to accept that prior prescribing has been less than economic and agree to institute changes as suggested by the health authorities professional advisers
• to justify prior prescribing and defend the clinical freedom to prescribe as one sees fit.

These two strategies are not, of course, mutually exclusive. The best possible defence against the accusation of profligacy in prescribing is a demonstration that one's prescribing does, indeed, achieve its clinical objectives. This is difficult in most instances and impossible in some, and the best one can do in most cases is demonstrate that one has made efforts to review one's prescribing and has made some attempt to review its cost effectiveness.

There are several ways of conducting a review of prescribing and then several possible ways forward with prescribing following such a review. If one can show improvement in respect of either generic prescribing, or prescribing in accordance with a formulary, this at least shows willingness to comply with the new drive for cost effectiveness. Clear demonstration that one's prescribing is in line with guidelines which others have determined (preferably on the basis of research) is indirect evidence that the clinical benefits are being pursued.

Reviewing current prescribing practice, using PACT

Reviewing current prescribing patterns is a form of audit in which data is collected on what is going on; this is compared to some standard or preconceived notion of what things should be like; and, if there is a mismatch between observed and expected, appropriate changes are instituted. This process is greatly facilitated in the UK by the availability of PACT data and other similar systems, since this spares the effort of data collection. (However, the information in PACT will usually need to be supplemented in order to be interpreted properly.) There are several possible approaches to PACT data: either begin by identifying high cost areas and tackle these first (this is the approach anticipated by the designers of PACT) or go through the data, therapeutic group by therapeutic group, in an order determined by the practice.

PACT data highlights several aspects of prescribing any one of which may be used as a starting point for review of prescribing (see Chapter 8):
- particular drugs which are costing the most (found in the 20 leading cost drugs on page 2 of the report)
- generic prescribing rates and how these compare with local averages
- previous year figures and the breakdown between those dispensed generically against those prescribed with proprietary (the data are found on page 3)
- particular therapeutic sub-groups which are costing the most (pages 6 and 7)
- therapeutic groups costing the most (page 2), or in which the largest number of items are being prescribed (page 3) or which groups are associated with the greatest cost per item suggesting the use of expensive drugs (page 5)
- proportions of new drug being used in particular therapeutic groups (page 2)
- time trends for cost for each therapeutic group (page 5), or for number of items (page 3) or cost per item (page 4), although in the case of the latter one can only look at this year versus last year whereas for cost one can see how things have varied over the previous 2 years.

However, with the exception of the top 20 drugs by cost category (page 2), the standard report can really only raise questions about prescribing—it cannot answer them. To gain more detailed understanding of what accounts for non-average aspects of prescribing, the more detailed Prescribing Catalogue will be needed. Fortunately, this can be ordered from the PPA piecemeal according to focus. Because the Catalogue gives so much detail it allows clear identification of what is driving prescribing costs, even allowing identification of single patients who are on unusual drugs or individual doctors' prescribing costs.

With a Prescribing Catalogue for a particular therapeutic area, it becomes possible to identify the most favoured drugs in use—individual preparations that are, perhaps, unduly expensive or are now viewed as obsolete. This sort of information might prompt a practice to begin to devise a formulary (see below). It also gives indications of 'spread' of prescribing which again might prompt the practice to restrict the range of drugs to be used for a therapeutic area.

The alternative approach, more typical of audit elsewhere, is to use PACT to review therapeutic areas which are chosen by the practice. Practitioners should examine their drug management for conditions in that therapeutic area and agree practice policies, at least about the drugs and pharmaceutical preparations they 'ought' to use. A PACT Prescribing Catalogue should then allow comparison of observed prescribing against the pattern that would be expected if the policy agreed were being operated. For example, a practice might decide to look at their prescribing for respiratory disease. In this area the main clinical condition to which prescribing relates is asthma. Thus the practice might discuss management of asthma and, ideally, ought to do this in relation to consensus such as the British Thoracic Society guidelines (British Thoracic Society, 1993).

They might also bear in mind the Audit Commission's report on Improving Prescribing and particularly its comments about the use of dry powder devices which they describe as 'premium price' preparations (Audit Commission, 1994). If this were done the practice might decide its practice policy is broadly in line with BTS guidelines. If this were the case the prescribing pattern emerging in the respiratory therapeutic group would show a relatively high proportion of inhaled steroids to ß-agonists (the Audit Commission appear to suggest a figure of 1.7 : 1 to be good practice); and it would show a relatively low use of dry powder devices and a low use of oral ß-agonists (which are pharmacologically much inferior to any inhaled form).

PACT Prescribing Catalogue can be used to generate these measures of prescribing and any shortfall relative to the target figures is material for discussion and action to improve. This is more typical of how the audit cycle works. A further advantage of this approach is that, in addition to identifying areas where prescribing could be cheaper, it also highlights areas of prescribing that are in line with expectation and may need to be defended against challenge by the health authority.

Defending prescribing in the face of a challenge

The thrust of the NHS reforms as they relate to prescribing in general practice is that doctors are being required to accept a degree of financial as well as clinical responsibility for their prescribing. While this will first impact on doctors with the arrival of PACT data and budget statements, these reports do not, of themselves, require any change from the prescribing doctor. What is more likely to prompt change is a visit of a prescribing adviser from the health authority. This might be a routine visit and part of a programme of visit to all practices in the area and may pose no particular threat or require no particular action on the part of the practice. It might be a visit prior to setting a budget, in which case the practice should prepare a case for having their budget maximized. However, it might be a visit to challenge the practice on the cost effectiveness of its prescribing. In this latter case, the practice should have anticipated such a visit, since it can be expected if any part of one's prescribing figures deviate from local norms or from expectations set in the budget.

The practice needs to be armed with information additional to PACT, which the health authority adviser will have already seen and probably analysed in great detail, with which to defend prescribing practice (Bradley, 1991). The kind of information that is useful to have in this circumstance is information to show how the practice population has higher morbidity than would be predicted on the basis of its age–sex mix. Practices with many elderly people would be advised to have figures for the proportions of those in rest homes and nursing homes, as these usually constitute the more frail elderly who need more care and more medication.

High cost prescribers for asthma medication might be able to make a case on the basis of an asthma register showing higher than average prevalence of asthma, combined with audit data on, say hospital admissions for asthma, which might show that the high cost of community care is accruing savings on hospital care and is associated with less morbidity in the community (e.g. days off school; days off work, etc.). High users of SSRI antidepressants may need to have data to show how the patients being so treated had higher than average suicide risk, or had previously been tried but failed to respond to tricyclics, or were unsuitable candidates for alternative antidepressants.

The first step in any defence against a challenge to prescribing is self-examination to avoid prescribing that is incontrovertibly wasteful (such as extensive use of peripheral or cerebral vasodilators) and, ideally, encouraging co-operation with existing directives such as having a high level of generic prescribing. The second step is having the appropriate clinical data, in as much case-by-case detail as possible, to make it clear that more costly prescribing is being associated with more clinical benefit. The lack of patient-related data is the great weakness in the PACT data available to the authority.

Drug formularies

A formulary is a list of drugs from which prescribers are expected to select the drugs they will use. In different settings and at different times the use of the word has varied in the extent to which it is used to describe a prescriptive or a voluntary list of medicaments (Lumley and Wells, 1992). Before the advent of the NHS, prescribing under the National Insurance schemes was regulated by local formularies. In 1927 the BMA and the Retail Pharmacists Union compiled a national formulary to serve doctors working under the National Insurance Act.

The *National War Formulary* was developed from this earlier formulary, but was more selective because of the scarcity of some ingredients and the need to exercize maximum economy at a time of crisis. It was from the *National War Formulary* that the *British National Formulary* (BNF) was developed, although it became less prescriptive and more advisory and began to contain much more additional information about the drugs besides their names and available formulations. With time, the number of drugs included in the BNF has grown such that the numbers are too great for it to be the basis of a list in the more recent sense. Nowadays the word formulary in general practice is used to mean a preferred list of drugs which doctors voluntarily commit themselves to using in preference to other drugs available.

The rationale for developing such a preferred drugs list is that by selecting a few of the many drugs available doctors are protected from the dangers of information overload. Patients are thus protected from accidental misuse. It has been discovered that most doctors tend to prescribe for most of the time from a fairly narrow range of drugs anyway (what has been referred to as their 'natural formulary') and developing a formulary is a rational extension of these habits (Bradley, 1990). However, formulary development can go much further in enhancing doctors' prescribing practice if it adopts recommended guidelines. The currently recommended method for construction involves the four steps of:

- establishing the criteria for the selection of drugs
- getting the target group of doctors to work cohesively to choose drugs for common conditions in general practice
- implementing the preferred list
- reviewing compliance with the preferred list.

Doctors involved are thus much more aware of the drugs they are prescribing, their pharmacology and therapeutic uses, why some should be preferred and why others should not be prescribed. Additional benefits are that implementation of a formulary will usually mean a switch to generic prescribing, because any preferred list that attempts to be short and based on considerations of cost effectiveness will, in nearly all instances, prefer generic names for drugs. It will also limit the introduction of new drugs, until they are evaluated. This improves safety for patients and reduces need for early information about new drugs.

A reduction in prescribing costs is a usual, though not inevitable, consequence of the introduction of a formulary. However, it is asserted by major proponents of formularies in general practice that cost savings should be seen as fortuitous rather than central (Reilly, 1992). This is important as prescribing advisers, who are more particularly focused on prescribing costs, promote formularies in the expectation that they will result in cost containment and may be disappointed if this is not seen to ensue. However, to have a formulary in place and implement it is a fairly solid defence to challenges to one's prescribing cost if they should escalate.

There are now many examples of formularies that have been developed by groups of GPs in different parts of the UK. Among the better known ones are the *Newcastle Formulary* (published by Oxford University Press), the *Northern Ireland Formulary* and the *Lothian Formulary* (Grant *et al.*, 1990; RCGP Northern Ireland Faculty, 1993; Lothian Liaison Committee, 1989). Formularies come in two basic formats. Some, such as the *Newcastle Formulary*, list the drugs under the conditions they are used to treat. Others, such as the *Northern Ireland Formulary* and indeed the BNF, list drugs by therapeutic class (usually related to the bodily system, e.g. cardiovascular or respiratory).

As well as listing the drugs and their normal formulations and dosages, many formularies will offer additional guidance on the use of the drugs or the management of the clinical conditions concerned. However, virtually all those involved in the production of these general practice formularies concede that the principal benefit of formulary construction is to those who develop the formulary; it is of more limited value to those who pick it up off the shelf (Lumley and Wells, 1992; Reilly, 1992). Therefore, the best advice to prescribers is to construct their own formulary with practice colleagues (if in group practice) and go through all the stages of formulary development as described below. This effort will be highly illuminating in terms of the use of drugs and of the therapeutic beliefs and practices of colleagues. This process should also bring about firmer commitment to whatever formulary is devised.

However, some of the effort involved in development can be spared by using the existing published formularies as a starting point or guide. The use of a good up-to-date formulary developed by other GPs with expert help may also be used to obviate the need to recruit specialist help to your own formulary group. The debate around selection can be made more efficient by discussing whether your group are for or against the published formulary drugs, with an obligation placed on anyone who wishes to add a drug not on the published formulary to make a case for it.

Formularies are not, however, a panacea for ensuring that all prescribing is truly rational and cost effective. How effective the formulary is in ensuring an improvement in prescribing and a closer link between prescribing and health gain, depends on how and by whom the formulary was developed, how many drugs are in the formulary, how well these cover common conditions, and the commitment of the doctors to its implementation. Thus a formulary which simply lists the doctors' preferred drugs or 'natural formulary' might not achieve the potential improvement in prescribing, particularly if some of the preferred drugs are obsolete, ineffective, relatively unsafe or unnecessarily expensive.

There is a need to have some expert input to the formulary development process, if only via existing published formularies. Ideally the selection of drugs for the formulary should be based on sound evidence of safety, efficacy, appropriateness, and economy. The formulary should also be selective: a target figure for the number of drugs which should cover over 90% of general practice prescribing is between 100 and 150 (Grant *et al.*, 1985). Fewer drugs than this would almost certainly not cover all common situations and so would lead to frequent breaches of the formulary guidance and gradually a lack of respect for the formulary. A number of drugs greater than 150 begins to defeat several purposes of the formulary, which might then be relegated to a reference source in competition with the BNF: a competition the BNF would easily win.

Finally, formulary development is most beneficial in largish (more than four doctors) group practices and is much less justifiable for a single-handed practitioner. It would not be valuable for the single-handed doctor to expend a lot of time and energy on formulary development when he or she is the only one likely to benefit. However, regular comparison of his or her prescribing, as evidenced by PACT, against a published formulary would go some way towards achieving many of the goals of formulary development.

How to develop a formulary

Reilly (1992) describes the process of formulary development as involving three main tasks. The first is to develop appropriate criteria for choosing medicines to be included in the formulary. How many medicines are in the formulary and whether or not they are the best that could be included is crucially dependent on these selection criteria. The basic criteria he suggests for selection are derived from the definition of rational prescribing proffered by Parish (1973). These state that the drug should be safe, effective, economic and appropriate to the patient's condition and acceptable to the patient.

To put these into operation, Reilly (1992) suggests each drug under consideration be profiled with regard to such factors as:

• the aim (in use) of the drug
• any observations about its use
• any drug or non-drug alternatives to the proposed drug
• the duration of therapy
• the metabolism of the drug
• any interactions
• the route and dosage usually used
• any adverse reactions there are, and how acceptable or otherwise are these to patients with the relevant condition.

By profiling the drug in this detailed way, drugs competing for a place on the formulary can be compared to each other and those with the most acceptable profile are accepted.

Even with all this effort made to chose between different drugs, one also needs to have a mind's eye view of how many drugs are required in each category. As a ballpark figure the number of drugs in each therapeutic sub-group tends to vary between one and five, with two or three being the most common number. The task is to get agreement among the doctors to operate the formulary.

Reilly (1992) describes practices going through a series of steps in undergoing this change in prescribing habit, which may amount to a major culture shift for some. The change required to operate the formulary will only occur, he argues, if the practice already works closely together and everyone feels and is actually involved in decision making. The final task is to ensure that the formulary works properly alongside other systems in the practice particularly the repeat prescription system.

Prescribing protocols and guidelines

As mentioned above, another buttress against challenge from the authority is to have in place some form of prescribing guidelines or prescribing policy. Such policies or guidelines have additional benefits in terms of reducing the potential for confusion between different doctors treating the same patient and they can help ensure that patients are consistently receiving the very best care that medical knowledge can offer. Ideally, guidelines should relate to the commonly presenting clinical conditions and should encompass all aspects of management including prescribing.

This is more logical than the formulary idea which, by giving so much prominence to the drugs, may reinforce the philosophy of 'a pill for every ill'. Thus in developing management guidelines one might begin with a condition such as diabetes. The guidelines might cover such issues as how the condition is to be diagnosed, what standard of evidence is to be required for a diagnosis, and what variants of the conditions there are. This might then lead to a series of sub-sets of guidelines for each of these various clinical manifestations of the condition; within each of these there would be guidance on what non-drug management is required, and then guidance on which drugs are to be preferred and under what circumstances each is the preferred option. Guidance should then be offered on what monitoring is required with regard to the future progress of the illness and with regard to possible adverse effects of the treatment. Guidelines of this calibre will have built into them both a formulary and prescribing policies such as a preference for generic prescribing except where this is not clinically appropriate.

There has been much research on the implementation of clinical guidelines and several important points have emerged (Grimshaw and Russell, 1993). Firstly, if guidelines are to be widely implemented they ought to be evidence based and not, as is often the case, based purely on consensus. That is to say they should be based on properly conducted research which, in many instances, will mean a randomized controlled trial (RCT) or a review of a series of RCTs conducted according to the guidance published by the Cochrane Collaboration (Chalmers *et al.*, 1985).

Consensus is acceptable so long as it is arrived at by a properly conducted consultation process (such as the Delphi technique) and the parties to the consensus have reviewed systematically whatever evidence is available according to the recognized guidelines on appraising evidence. Guidelines also need to be locally developed and locally owned. This may seem, initially, to be contradictory or, at least, impractical as each local guidelines development group cannot be expected to systematically review all the research evidence in relation to every possible clinical problem. This would indeed be a tremendous waste of effort. The best way to marry the need for guidelines to be both locally owned and to be evidence based is for the local group to take an existing set of evidence-based guidelines, check them for the rigour with which they were complied (as was suggested for drug formularies) and then modify them to take account of local circumstances. Thus while the evidence-based consensus guidelines might say that long term glucose control should be monitored using haemoglobin A_1 concentration, local laboratory facilities may mean that this has to be done using fructosamine. The similarity between this process and that of formulary construction is obvious. The process, if properly conducted, is profoundly educational. However, similar problems with implementation also occur.

A term that is sometimes used synonymously with 'guidelines' is 'protocols'. Although it may seem a trifle pedantic, it is worth stressing the subtle but important distinction between these two terms. The word protocol implies something that is a good deal more prescriptive than a guideline. There is a desire on the part of some segments of health services management to have the nature and content of the service to patients more closely specified and, ultimately, monitored in a highly specific and tight way. Thus a prescribing protocol would specify the drugs to be used in the treatment of any given clinical condition and any prescribing outside the protocol would be seen as a breach of the protocol and, presumably, investigated in some fairly censorious manner.

This approach to the control of prescribing is clearly much more vigorously challenging to clinical freedom and is, naturally, resisted by clinicians when this significance of protocols comes to be appreciated. Some would content that this is too sinister a view of protocols but it does highlight, perhaps caricature, the distinction between guidelines and protocols and clarifies why, for clinicians at least, guidelines are greatly to be preferred (McCormick, 1994).

Repeat prescribing

As well as addressing issues of choice of drug, prescribing policies are needed to tackle other aspects of the prescribing process such as how long the drug is to be prescribed, under what conditions will drugs be stopped or changed, and what checks are in place to ensure the patient is receiving and taking the drug as prescribed and is not encountering either side effects or lack of efficacy. These issues are particularly pertinent where the prescribing is for medications which are to be taken long term. Such long term prescribing is dealt with in a variety of ways in different healthcare systems, but within the UK system they are generally dealt with within a 'repeat prescribing' system. A repeat prescribing system is a mechanism within a practice which enables a patient to obtain medicines he or she needs either long term or recurrently without the need to consult with the doctor each time a further supply is required. Such a system strives to ensure that patients obtain the medicines they need without burdening the doctors with clinically unjustified consultations while still retaining some degree of control and monitoring of the patient's medicines use. Sometimes this sort of prescribing without face-to-face contact between doctor and patient is referred to as 'indirect prescribing' (Reilly, 1985) although this term also encompasses prescribing for acute presentations without face-to-face contact. Clearly repeat prescribing is a strategy employed mostly to deal with the management of long term prescribing but it is not entirely synonymous with repeat prescribing either as sometimes prescriptions are repeated at face to face contacts. Figure 9.1 shows how the three terms, 'repeat prescribing', 'indirect prescribing', and 'long term prescribing' are overlapping rather than synonymous. Harris and Dajda (1996) have argued that repeat prescribing be defined as prescribing done using the repeat prescribing facility of GP computer systems, but he also admits that this rather tautologous definition does not fully encompass what is commonly understood by the term 'repeat prescribing' in UK general practice which is where the phenomenon (almost uniquely) occurs.

Fig. 9.1 *Relationship between repeat prescribing, long-term prescribing, and indirect prescribing*

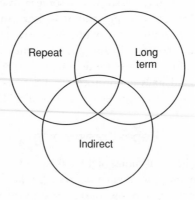

Zermansky (1996) has divided repeat prescribing into three components, each of which require the practice to have a mechanism and policy in place. He sees the process as consisting of

- the production of repeat prescriptions, which he sees as largely an administrative task
- the management of the repeat prescribing which he sees as a task for the practice management
- the exertion of clinical control which he, naturally, sees as the responsibility of the doctors.

The administrative task is usually delegated to receptionists. It deals with how patients are allowed to make requests (must they be made in person or can they be made by telephone, post, fax, etc.) and what will be done following the request to ensure that an appropriate prescription form is generated and then signed by the doctor, and how that form will be transmitted on to the patient or, in some cases, directly to the pharmacy. The administrative policies need to clarify other issues such as whether or not clinical records are made available routinely—we would suggest this is generally good practice—and how quickly requests will be turned around—we would suggest practices should aim for 1–2 working days maximum. Consideration should also be given to what information will be provided to patients to help them understand and use the system effectively. This is often done in the practice leaflet but there is merit in having a special leaflet on the repeat prescribing system specifically.

The management task involves ensuring there are mechanisms in place to deal with

- the possibility of patients seeking medicine they are not authorized to have without face-to-face contact
- patients who overuse or underuse their medicines
- patients who do not attend when they are due to be seen for review and hence are seeking medicines after the interval which has been decided for their going without face-to-face contact
- ensuring that all these misuses of the system by patients are drawn to the attention of prescribers.

The system will also need to be able to deal with urgent requests for essential medicines within a shorter time frame that the normal one for the system (such as urgent requests for inhalers for asthma) and have some means of gradually escalating pressure on patients to force them to be seen when due without actually obliging the patient to run out of medicine in order to generate a consultation.

The clinical task involves the usual matters of ensuring that

- each drug is clinically justified
- drugs which interact are avoided where possible and suitable precautions are taken where interacting drugs are unavoidable in combination
- a review date is set appropriate to the patient's clinical condition and the requirement for monitoring the therapy
- crucially, that the patient is given sufficient information to enable him or her to understand the purpose of the medicine, the need for its continuance (if this is the case), the conditions under which it may be stopped, altered or substituted and how and when further supplies are to be obtained and when and how a review consultation will be set up.

Issues of drug choice are dealt with in Chapters 5 and 6 and the issue of prescription length is also dealt with in Chapter 6. The purpose of treatment needs to be clarified and, in the context of repeat prescribing, this relates to whether the drug is being prescribed for an acute, recurrent, or long-term condition. In the case of acute conditions repeat, or indeed indirect, prescribing is not usually appropriate. In the case of recurrent conditions it is probably best to prescribe directly face to face until the variability of medication need is gauged and the average need over time can be reasonably well established. In the case of more stable chronic conditions repeat prescribing of fixed quantities can usually be established fairly early and review may be carried out in relation to the known pattern of the disease or the perceived risk of the appearance of either side effects or diminution of efficacy of the prescribed treatment. Usually, this is understood to involve at least annual review. It is also worth considering at the outset of repeat prescribing whether the treatment is disease-modifying or primarily symptomatic. In the latter case, it is important this is made clear to the patient when the repeat prescription is being set up as the physician is much more likely to want to stop symptomatic treatments if other conditions for which disease-modifying treatment is required supervene. The potential risks of the drug either alone or in combination with other drugs may also lead to a need to establish more frequent review even where the clinical condition does not require such close review. Likewise, drugs with a propensity to induce dependence, while not usually recommended for repeat prescribing, may, under certain circumstance be prescribed on repeat but, in this case, closer review would be recommended. Finally, drugs which are expensive, even only moderately so, should usually be prescribed in smaller quantities and hence at shorter intervals because of the greater risk of waste if they are not used. Table 9.1 indicates how repeat prescribing should be modified according to the purpose of treatment, the duration of treatment and the nature of the drug(s).

Table 9.1 *Modification of repeat prescribing policy according to anticipated duration of treatment, purpose of treatment and type of drug*

Type of treatment	Anticipated duration of treatment		
	Acute	Chronic stable	Chronic relapsing/ recurrent
Symptomatic— safe drug	Avoid repeating	Long repeat (3–6 months)	Establish pattern first, then long repeat
Symptomatic— unsafe/expensive drug	Avoid repeating	Repeat at intervals related to risks/ monitoring	Short interval repeats
Disease modifying— safe drug	Avoid repeating	Long repeat (3–6 months)	Establish pattern first, then long repeat
Disease modifying— unsafe/expensive drug	Avoid repeating	Repeat at intervals related to risks/ monitoring	Short interval repeats

Naturally, all of the above points need to be considered in the context of the individual patient and the final regimen for treatment, its monitoring and review, and the repeat prescribing interval should, ideally, be negotiated and agreed with the patient. Thus the patient's age, intelligence, degree of social support, known or suspected reliability about complying and so on will need to be considered. Furthermore, patients should be informed on all points regarding the purpose, duration, and safety of his or her treatment.

Research on repeat prescribing suggests that it is extremely common, with one study (Harris and Dajda, 1996) suggesting it accounts for 75% of items prescribed and 81% of drug costs although their definition is, perhaps, questionable (see above). Other studies (National Audit Office, 1993; Audit Commission, 1994; Purves and Kennedy, 1994) concur that repeat prescribing may account for about two thirds of all prescribing and three quarters of prescribing costs. Zermansky's (1996) evaluation of repeat prescribing systems in 50 Leeds practices suggested that there are considerable deficiencies in the control of repeat prescribing in many practices, with breakdowns in clinical control appearing to be the most common problem, although Taylor (1996) suggests that this may be in part a problem of record keeping by doctors. It is clearly an area that needs some attention and is likely to become an area subjected to increasing scrutiny by health services managers. (Bradley, 1996) Standards have been suggested for repeat prescribing, two of which are reproduced in Boxes 9.1 and 9.2.

Box 9.1 *Ten requirements of a good repeat prescribing system*

Patient able to get one in 24 hours
Meticulous accuracy
Clear but flexible recall system
Clear record of patient's drugs what on and when last supplied
Cost efficient and user friendly
Built in quality assurance
Means of checking compliance
All prescriptions reviewed and signed by a doctor who knows the patient and has the notes
Flexible to meet patient needs
Drugs supplied ordered by a doctor and reviewed on a regular basis

(Source: Medical Advisers Support Centre, as cited by National Audit Office, 1993)

Primary–secondary care issues

One of the paradoxical effects of the indicative prescribing scheme was to make more explicit something which had been an implicit feature of the system for some time. In the 'Improving Prescribing' document introducing the IPS, the

---

Box 9.2 *Features of the ideal repeat prescribing system*

Information

- what the patient is on
- what they are for
- how often to be seen
- what is being monitored
- whether due; not yet due or overdue
- authorized to have or needs to see the doctor

Other features

- flexible and efficient
- accommodates reasonable expectations
- accommodates unscheduled requests for essential medicines
- escalates the pressure to be seen
- delivers within one working day
- detects non-attenders
- clearly understood by all staff and patients

(Source: Bradley, 1993)

Government's commitment that no patient should be denied necessary medicine was reiterated. However, it was also made clear that one of the means for fulfilling this commitment was that the budget for prescribing in the Family Health Service was to remain open-ended (Department of Health, 1990). In other words, should more money be spent than was anticipated, the government was prepared to return to Parliament and have additional monies voted to cover the costs.

This special budgetary arrangement, which had already existed, was retained but was also highlighted. This became increasingly widely known to the secondary sector whose entire budget, inclusive of the drugs element, was cash-limited. Inevitably, doctors and finance managers in the secondary care sector saw the obvious implication that anything which could not be afforded in the hospital could still be prescribed and paid for as long as the GP would take on prescribing. It was already well established that if a hospital doctor prescribes a drug for a patient returning to the community and that drug is needed longer term then the GP would continue prescribing of that drug.

There were also existing guidelines on how this should be handled between primary and secondary care, but these were rather vague, implying that such practice was acceptable so long as both doctors agreed to it. The issue of who carried responsibility for the prescribing was not made too explicit and the medical defence organizations, while agreeing that the doctor who wrote the prescription carried some responsibility, maintained that the exact proportioning of responsibility was something not yet established by sufficient case law.

As the loophole became clearer to hospitals they began to try to shift prescribing costs with greater and greater frequency, and to push this further by stopping or severely curtailing the prescribing done at their out-patients and by limiting the drugs supplied to patients on discharge. The practice even began of hospitals who wanted patients to have drugs not available on their increasingly restrictive formularies asking GPs to initiate patients on these new drugs, sometimes even while the patient was still in hospital.

All these attempts to ask the GP to take on additional prescribing came at a difficult time for GPs, who, although they did not have budgets *per se*, were beginning to experience something akin to the financial constraints that their hospital colleagues had lived with for some time. Tensions naturally arose to the extent that the Government had to issue, in 1991, revised guidelines on prescribing across the secondary–primary care interface.

These new guidelines, without denying that the arrangements were ultimately up to the clinicians concerned (EL91/127), were much more explicit about who bore prescribing responsibility, placing it squarely on the shoulders of the doctor who wrote the prescription. In so doing the hope was, we would surmise, to urge GPs to stand up more firmly to hospital consultants and to refuse to take on this responsibility for what were increasingly often high-tech and high-cost drugs.

The effect on containing the increasing pressure to shift prescribing responsibility and costs to primary care was rather limited and evidence of so-called 'cost shifting' continued to accumulate. By 1994 the government was forced to act again (EL94/72) and this time a range of drugs of this high-tech, high-cost nature was taken out of the primary care sector and responsibility for prescribing them and paying for them was taken back into hospitals who were to be given extra resources to allow for this.

In 1996 a new challenge to these arrangements arrived in the form of ß-interferon for the treatment of multiple sclerosis (Walley and Barton, 1995). This is a very expensive treatment (cost £10 000 p.a. per patient) which seems to provide some benefit in terms of relapse prevention in only a proportion of multiple sclerosis suffers, specifically those with the form of the disease known as relapsing–remitting multiple sclerosis. The government once again had to act with the issue of a further EL (EL95/97) urging health authorities to control access to this treatment and advising against primary care prescribing. The NHS Executive in each region and local health authorities moved quickly to establish local arrangements to control the use of this treatment and provide funding for it to the secondary sector. In all instances (to our knowledge) they have advised against primary care prescribing and indeed any prescribing unless part of a clinical trial.

Clearly, this sort of shuffling of responsibility for prescribing and its cost between the primary and secondary care is not very satisfactory, least of all for patients. Much hope is being placed on the fact that the authorities responsible for both primary and secondary care are now united and hold responsibility for both primary and secondary care prescribing budgets.

How this advantage will be exploited remains to be seen. In the meantime, what ought doctors to do? The first and most important thing is that they should come together and discuss such matters. Part of the problem over the past few years has been change in policy occurring in both primary and secondary care independent of each other but with major impact on the other sector. This has happened both ways with GPs, in response to their budgetary pressures, refusing to go along with hospital recommendations about therapy, but without conferring with the hospital.

Through dialogue we should be able to change the current practice referred to as 'cost shifting' with its implications of blame attribution, to one of 'cost sharing' in which we both recognize that we each have budgets and we have a common goal of making sure that our shared patients get the best care that can be got out of that limited budget. The concept of non cash-limited budget in primary care is an illusion, as all that happens if primary care gets voted more money for drugs via the special arrangements referred to above is that there is less money available to the whole NHS for the following year and so other treatments become unavailable. By talking to one another we can come up with what have been referred to as 'effective shared care guidelines'.

Effective shared care guidelines

Effective shared care guidelines should become the definitive statement on how care is to be shared between hospital and general practice. Shared care guidelines need to define areas of responsibility and which aspects of care will be exclusively the responsibility of the hospital, which aspects of care will be exclusively the responsibility of the GP, and, where there is no such exclusivity of responsibility, specification of when and how one party will assume responsibility and when and how responsibility will be transferred back to the other party to the agreement.

While these have been developed in respect of some important disease areas, such as for patients on renal dialysis, increasingly they will need to be developed for a host of conditions for which care is shared across the primary–secondary care interface. They should, in the longer term, become increasingly patient specific.

This process clearly all depends on good and close communication between hospital and practice and effective shared care guidelines should be explicit about how and when such communication will be effected. Thus, for instance, the hospital, ideally, ought to provide a 24 hour telephone contact number for GPs to get guidance on aspects of patient management that may present as an emergency. Furthermore, a clinical summary of the case needs to be sent to the GP (e.g. by fax), prior to the patient's arriving at the practice requesting a further supply of medicine recommended by the hospital. This summary should contain, in addition to the information on the drug, information about the disease or its treatment if the disease is not one could expect most GPs to know something about.

With regard to the drug, as much information as possible needs to be given to GPs who will, if they prescribe it, be taking full legal and moral responsibility for the effects of the drug. As a minimum, the drug information should indicate

- whether or not the drug is been recommended for use within the terms of its Produce Licence
- the drug's therapeutic classification
- dose and route for administration
- adverse reactions known or likely to occur (including their incidence, identification, and management)
- any clinically relevant drug interactions and their management
- any additional information the GP or patient ought to know in order to use the drug safely (e.g. storage information).

Other elements of a shared care package should be, to whatever degree is appropriate, individualized to the particular patient. It is also highly desirable that such individualized guidelines or treatment plans would have the patient's and GP's full and informed consent. Such guidelines need to be documented and kept readily available in practices for ready reference when facing a patient, although this is not a substitute for written invidualized information for doctor and patient when the repeat prescription is being issued for the first time.

Such guidelines will not resolve all financial difficulties and may even result in either primary or secondary care providers or even both having to go back to the authority to argue for additions to their budgets. It will also eventually lead to both parties having to agree that not all that they want for their patients can be provided within available resources and so criteria for resource allocation (or rationing) will have to be agreed. At least, though, under these unpalatable circumstances, the clinicians involved will know that they have worked together for the good of patients and that they are getting the best available from limited resources.

Managed care and disease management

The preceding part of this chapter describes current ways in which doctors might adapt, and it seems are adapting, to the new NHS. However, the changes to the NHS will not stop at PACT and the indicative prescribing scheme. One of the more significant recent proposals is that of disease management which is one aspect of the slightly broader concept of 'managed care' (Panton *et al.*, 1995).

Managed care can be defined as 'a process of healthcare delivery which integrates elements of access, quality and cost', where the provider delivery system is managed through the contracting and service specification process with the aim of improving efficiency. Disease management is a process where 'all those responsible for prevention, diagnosis, and treatment of disease agree to the standards, personnel and cost by which care will be provided'.

Agreed systems for diagnosis and treatment are inherent in the concept of disease management, with clinical guidelines, or sometimes protocols, as a cornerstone. Thus disease management (DM) moves away from a focus on control of individual costs (e.g. for drugs) towards a consideration of total costs of management. For the NHS this means the possibility of taking into account potential secondary care costs as well as those incurred in primary care.

These are concepts that were developed in the US, and, while they may not be immediately applicable to the NHS now, there is intense interest in them within the Department of Health (DoH) and growing pressure from the pharmaceutical industry to be allowed to develop them in the UK. Health authorities have been in discussion with pharmaceutical companies about the possible development of disease management schemes in the UK. The NHS Executive have been forced to adopt a holding position effectively banning further development for the time being.

Some of the elements of managed care have been in place in some parts of the NHS for years. Proactive management of prescribing issues has occurred in the hospital sector, via clinical pharmacy services, since the 1970s and 1980s. In primary care generic prescribing, formulary development and feedback to prescribers (via PACT reports, FHSA professional advisers and educational outreach) exist to varying degrees already.

The use of clinical guidelines to articulate standards of care fits well with the drive towards evidence-based practice. Such guidelines might range from preventive strategies (e.g. lifestyle advice), through self-medication (e.g. antacids), investigations (e.g. *H. pylori* testing) and further treatment (drugs, surgery). Monitoring and audit, also being actively promoted throughout the health service, are essential parts of the process.

A feature of managed care programmes is their requirement for 'prior authorization' of prescribing of costly drugs, particularly those which have been recently introduced. Although the NHS may not yet have introduced prior authorization, it is starting to address the managed introduction of new drugs, planning for the clinical and financial implications. Purchasers are playing a lead role in this respect and are increasingly prepared to advise their providers.

The development of enhanced Drug and Therapeutics Committees to provide advice across both primary and secondary care is an important further innovation for the late 1990s. Supported by high-level drug information input, such committees will direct their advice to support GPs in critical analysis of new pharmaceutical products. The first such committees are already established in Scotland and the West Midlands of England (Bradley, 1995a). Although concerns have been expressed at the already high level of prescribing advice to GPs (for example, through PACT and FHSA Professional Advisers) it is generally acknowledged that the introduction of new drugs is a key area where independent information is needed quickly (Bradley, 1995b).

Pharmacists and primary care prescribing

The 1990s have seen continuing developments in the input of pharmacists to the prescribing process. As we have already said, this role is well-established in the hospital setting both at macro level (input to drug policy through Drug and Therapeutics Committees) and micro level (advice to individual prescribers about individual patients' drug therapy).

In 1986 the Nuffield Inquiry into pharmacy identified that closer working relationships between GPs and their community pharmacist colleagues could benefit patients in a number of ways (Committee of Inquiry, Nuffield Foundation, 1986). This theme was taken up in the recommendations of the Joint Working Party Report (Pharmaceutical Care) in 1993 which identified the community pharmacists potential contribution in advice to GPs on prescribing.

The DoH provided £1 million in 1995 for pilot projects in 16 FHSAs to test differing models of community pharmacist prescribing advice. However, by this time there was already considerable activity, ranging from arrangements between individual community pharmacists and GPs to more ambitions educational outreach programmes involving community pharmacists.

Keele University's IMPACT programme began in 1994 using specially trained community pharmacists to deliver targeted information on prescribing to GPs. By 1996 the scheme was running in nine FHSAs and over 60 community pharmacists were involved. The University of Keele also launched an innovative clinical pharmacy service to GP practices in 1994, where a clinical pharmacist/clinical pharmacologist team provided tailored prescribing advice and prescribing audit. The theme of closer working between GPs and pharmacists is reflected in the emerging needs of patients arising from hospital discharge.

Nurse prescribing

The impetus for nurse prescribing came from the anomaly that district nurses and health visitors visited patients in their own homes but had to go through a wasteful process of returning to the surgery to obtain prescriptions for simple items such as wound dressings and basic medicines.

Following the Crown report in the 1980s, the nursing profession lobbied hard and successfully for prescribing rights for nurses with a district nurse or health visitor qualification (DoH, 1989). The initiative finally resulted in a series of eight 'demonstration' projects which began in autumn 1994 (Anon, 1994). A Nurse Prescribers' Formulary (NPF) was developed as an addendum to the BNF and provided the definitive list of what could be prescribed (see Box 9.3). Each prescription is issued on a special form according to protocols which cover initial assessment of the patient and subsequent review and tailoring of the treatment. In January 1995 six prescription-only items were added to the NPF. These were cadexomer-iodine, co-dantramer, mebendazole, miconazole, nystatin, and streptokinase. The other items in the NPF are available over the counter but are often prescribed by doctors, particularly for patients exempt from prescription charges.

Box 9.3 *Types of items included in the NPF*

Laxatives	Mild analgesics
Anaesthetics	Drugs for the mouth
Drugs for threadworms	Drugs for scabies and headlice
Skin preparations	Disinfection and cleansing products
Wound management products	Elastic hosiery
Urinary catheters and appliances	Stoma care products
Appliances and reagents for diabetes	Fertility and gynaecology products

---

Eligible nurses are obliged to undergo special training before being allowed to prescribe. They are encouraged to prescribe generically and for not more than a month at a time. When the nurse is directly employed by the practice, costs are attributed to the patient's GP and charged to the practice.

Nurse prescribing was initially restricted to eight evaluation sites, one in each of eight Regional Health Authority areas in England. The evaluation of nurse prescribing was subsequently extended by allowing it throughout an entire district (Bolton). In the 1996 White Paper, *Primay Care Delivering the Future*, the government promised to roll out the nurse prescribing scheme to a further seven NHS trusts in each of the remaining regions for further evaluation and expressed the intention to fully implement the scheme in due course (DoH, 1996).

Initial evaluation of nurse precribing has been very encouraging (Luker *et al.*, 1997). Nurses reported that being able to prescribe saved them time as they were no longer required to obtain presciptions from patients' GPs for items in the formulary. Nurses participating did admit to some initial anxieties about taking responsibilty for their own prescriptions, but this was compensated for by feelings of increased satisfaction, autonomy, and esteem. Doctors were also positive in their evaluations. They did not find cause to override the nurse's prescribing decisions and they were grateful to be relieved of the burden of prescribing items needed by nurses, particularly items such as wound care products about which GPs freely admitted nurses usually knew more than they did. Although patients in the pilot sites had had little experience of nurse prescribing, they were generally supportive of the development. Furthermore, many of the anticipated disadvantages of nurse prescribing did not seem to materialize. Thus nurses did not find it increased their workload, it did not impair their working relationship with other nursing colleagues unable to prescribe, and pressure to prescribe items which patients had previously been urged to buy for themselves was not reported. Finally, the concern that nurses might be inundated with attention from pharmaceutical company representatives was found not to be warranted, although this may yet occur as the number of nurses prescribing rises.

Critics of the scheme note that it is still limited to a relatively small proportion of nurses working in primary care, and limited to quite a restricted range of products. It has still not removed the phenomenon of nurses having to wait around for GPs to just ratify their prescribing decisions in areas of primary care involving complex therapies where nurses have now built up considerable expertise, such as family planning and chronic disease management. However, nurses, including those with the additional qualification required by nurse prescribing scheme, are not equipped by their basic training to undertake more complex aspects of diagnosis or therapeutics such as dealing with patients with multiple health problems. Such training cannot readily be provided as an 'add on' either, and so to extend the scheme beyond its current limitations might prove problematic. One proposal which might allow nurses to prescribe safely and effectively across a broader range of products, therapeutic areas, and patient groups is for them to work jointly with pharmacists. Such a development might be facilitated by the more flexible arrangements for primary care service provision envisaged in the Delivering the Future White Paper.

Private prescribing and the NHS

The inexorable rise of the prescription charge has brought with it increasing awareness among the public that many drugs cost less than the current charge. Two main methods of avoiding the NHS prescription charge have followed—purchasing the item over the counter (providing it is not a prescription only medicine) and issue of a private prescription where the medicine is a POM but will be cheaper than the charge.

The consumer organizations have been quick to point out the potential savings to the public, and the Consumers' Association in *Drug and Therapeutics Bulletin* has for some years published a list of medicines costing less than the prescription charge (Anon, 1993).

GPs have expressed concern about whether their terms of service permit the issue of a private prescription. The debate centres around the wording which currently states that the prescriber 'shall' order any necessary items on an NHS prescription. Clarification issued by the NHS Executive claimed that so long as the GP offered the patient the option of an NHS script, the spirit of the regulations would be met. However GPs have expressed concerns at this interpretation. Some have called for a change in the relevant wording, replacing 'shall' with 'might'.

The arguments about 'creeping privatization of the NHS' through this practice have focused on the principle of a right to an NHS prescription. Concern has also been expressed at the loss of prescribing data which would occur if the practice became widespread, since private prescriptions are not entered into PACT data. Arguably such a loss is occurring already with recommendations from GPs and pharmacists for patients to purchase items over the counter where this would be cheaper. Pharmacists are free to set their own fees for dispensing private prescriptions. Ethical requirements mean it is inappropriate to direct patients to a particular pharmacy to have their prescription dispensed, but many GPs find it useful to discuss costs of commonly written private prescriptions with local pharmacists.

Impact of information technology

Rapid developments in information technology have implications for both prescribers and patients. The launch of the electronic BNF on disk and CD-ROM in November 1995 marked the start of a new age of computerized prescribing support. Electronic systems will not be limited to the provision of information but will provide interactive decision support. The preliminary evaluation report of the NHS Executive's pilot project, PRODIGY, is not yet available. PRODIGY includes management and prescribing guidelines for over 60 common conditions, where the prescriber will be offered appropriate drug therapy choices from which a selection can be made.

The guidelines were developed by the Medical Advisers Support Centre (MASC) in consultation with the Royal Pharmaceutical Society and others. The GP has the option to override the alternatives suggested by the software, so flexibility is maintained. Nevertheless it is likely that PRODIGY and other future software have the potential to become a powerful influence on prescribing. Access to relevant associated information about drugs at the time of prescribing, especially from an independent and authoritative source, could help practitioners to reach prescribing decisions which are more overtly evidence-based.

Such software fulfils an educational function as well as its practical role. However the rate of adoption of systems such as PRODIGY will be dependent on its user-friendliness, access to appropriate hardware which can respond quickly to inputs, and the extent to which the software is seen to enhance practice in a way that meets GPs' needs.

Alongside these developments for health professionals, the public will have access to more information than ever before. Written information in patient packs will be the tip of the information iceberg. Electronic communication will offer the public the opportunity to access further information about medicines. Questions are already being asked about the independence and quality of such information. Health professionals will have to get used to the idea that no one 'owns' this information and must expect more questions from the public about their treatment.

References

Anon, (1993). Medicines cheaper over the counter. *Drug and Therapeutics Bulletin*, **31**(15), supplement.

Anon, (1994). Nurse prescribing 'demonstration' starts on October 3. *Pharmaceutical Journal*, **253**, 440.

Audit Commission (1994). *A prescription for improvement. Towards more rational prescribing in general practice.* HMSO, London.

Bradley, C. P. (1990). PACT: adviser suggests a DIY approach. *Mims Magazine* 15 November, 47–50.

Bradley, C. P. (1991). When the adviser call, what do you do? *Mims Magazine* 15 May, 53–5.

Bradley, C. (1993). Promoting practice services: prescribing. *Horizons* March, 115–17.

Bradley, C. P. (1995a). Do GPs need still more prescribing advice? *Prescriber* 19 October, 13–14.

Bradley, C. P. (1995b). New drugs: a challenge to the prescribing budget. *Prescriber* 5 November, 86–7.

Bradley, C. (1996). Repeat prescribing: do we need to clean up our act? *Prescriber* 5 December, 13.

British Thoracic Society (1993). Guidelines on the management of asthma. *Thorax*, **48** (Suppl), S1–24.

Chalmers, I., Enkin, M., Keirse, M. J. N. C. (1985). *Effective care in pregnancy and childbirth.* Oxford University Press, Oxford.

DoH (1990). *Improving prescribing.* HMSO, London.

DoH (1989). *Report of the advisory group on nurse prescribing* (Crown Report). Department of Health, London.

DoH (1996). *Primary care: delivering the future.* Stationery Office, London.

Grant, G. B., Gregory, D. A., van Zwanenberg, T. D. (1985). Development of a limited formulary for general practice. *Lancet*, **1**, 1030–1.

Grant, G. B., Gregory, D. A., van Zwanenberg, T. D. (1990). *A basic formulary of general practice*, 2nd edn. Oxford University Press, Oxford.

Grimshaw, J. M., Russell, I. T. (1993). Effect of clinical guidelines on medical practice: a systematic review of rigorous evaluations. *Lancet*, **342**, 1317–21.

Harris, C. M., Dajda, R. (1996). The scale of repeat prescribing. *British Journal of General Practice*, **46**, 649–53.

Lothian Liaison Committee (1989). *Lothian Formulary*, 2nd edn. Royal College of General Practitioners South East of Scotland Faculty, Edinburgh.

Luker, K., Austin, L., Ho, C., Ferguson, B., Smith. K. (1997). Nurse prescribing: the views of nurses and other healthcare professionals. *British Journal of Community Health Nursing*, **2**, 69–74.

Lumley P., Wells, F. (1992). Formularies and their use. In *Medicines: responsible prescribing*, ed. F. O. Wells. Queen's University Belfast, Belfast.

McCormick, J. (1994). The place of judgement in medicine. *British Journal of General Practice*, **44**, 50–1.

National Audit Office (1993). *Repeat prescribing by general medical practitioners in England*. HMSO, London.

Nuffield Foundation Committee of Inquiry (1986). *Pharmacy*. Nuffield Foundation, London.

Panton, R. S., Cox, I. G., Norwood, J. (1995). The development of managed care in the United Kingdom. *Pharmaceutical Journal*, **255**, 781–2.

Parish, P. A. (1973). Drug prescribing—the concern of all. *Royal Society of Health Journal*, **93**, 213–17.

Purves, I., Kennedy, J. (1994). *The quality of general practice repeat prescribing*. Sowerby Unit for Primary Care Informatics, Newcastle upon Tyne.

RCGP Northern Ireland Faculty (1993). *Practice Formulary*, 3rd edn. Royal College of General Practitioners Northern Ireland Faculty, Belfast.

Reilly, P. (1992). General practice formularies: advice on drafting and practice use. In *Medicines: responsible prescribing*, ed. F. O. Wells. Queen's University, Belfast.

Reilly, P. M. (1985). Repeat prescribing in a Belfast practice. MD Thesis, Queen's University, Belfast.

Taylor, R. J. (1996). Repeat prescribing—still our Achilles' heel? *British Journal of General Practice*, **46**, 640–641.

Walley, T., Barton, S. (1995). A purchaser perspective of managing new drugs: interferon beta as a case study. *British Medical Journal*, **311**, 796–9.

Zermansky, A. G. (1996). Who controls repeats? *British Journal of General Practice*, **46**, 643–7.

CHAPTER TEN

Non-prescription or over-the-counter medicines and the role of the pharmacist

Christine Bond and Colin Bradley

In the UK, the retail and wholesale dealings of all medicines and poisons are regulated primarily by the Medicines Act 1968, together with the Poisons Act 1972 and the Misuse of Drugs Act 1971. Sale and supply of medicines (by which is meant 'medicinal products' and includes any substance or article sold or supplied for administration to human beings or animals for a medicinal purpose) is controlled by the Part III of the Medicines Act 1968, and by orders made under it. The underlying principle is that a medicinal product may be sold only from a registered pharmacy under the supervision of a pharmacist, unless it is on the General Sales List (GSL) or is subject to some other exemptions under the Act, for example the Prescription Only Medicines List (POM). Any other medicine is known as a Pharmacy Medicine (P).

A strikingly similar position to that in the UK has evolved in other developed countries, although the US is unusual in that it has only two categories of medicines, equivalent to POM and GSL. However in practice, the actual sales distribution of individual medicines in the US closely follows the UK model and there is current lobbying to introduce a 'pharmacy only' category.

In the UK, any new drug entity gaining a medicine licence automatically has POM status. After 2 years, this status defaults to P unless there is a re-application to retain the POM status. In order to change this status subsequently, a formal application has to be made to the Medicines Control Agency (MCA). Evidence of safety and efficacy is central to this. The submissions are considered in detail by various committees, including representatives from relevant professional bodies. It is a time consuming and expensive process, in spite of a recent streamlining of the application procedure (Medicines Control Agency, 1992).

In 1987 the European Commission announced its intention to harmonize the distribution of medicines in Europe, with the intention of bringing consistency to the availability of medicines by either prescription or pharmacy sale. For the UK that would have resulted in the ingredients of some pharmacy medicines such as ephedrine, diphenhydramine, phenylpropanolamine, and codeine, moving to POM status. This would have had far-reaching implications for the industry, the NHS and the whole culture of self care. It was calculated (Baker, 1993) that £100 million sales would have been threatened. However, the proposals were reconsidered and approached from the pharmacy perspective, and the final decision was that 'no medicine should remain POM unless necessary for reasons of safety'. This became the European Community directive (1992) for medicines classification 92/26/CEE (see Box 10.1).

Box 10.1   *European community directive for medicines classification 92/26/CEE*

Medicines should be POM only if:
• they are dangerous if used other than under medical supervision
• they are frequently used incorrectly
• they are new and need further investigation
• they are normally administered by injection

The role of the community pharmacist

Several reports and publications (DoH, 1987; DoH, 1992; National Audit Office, 1992; Nuffield Foundation Committee of Enquiry, 1986) have recently emphasized the need for a greater involvement of the community pharmacist in primary healthcare. Pharmacists are highly trained health care professionals with a specific expertise in drugs, whose potential has been utilized in the hospital setting but currently is not fully realized in the community. Community pharmacists are expected to become more involved in the future in order to promote cost effective health care; that is, pharmaceutical care for patients will be both increased and extended.

Historically, the GP and community pharmacist have a common ancestor in the apothecary, an adviser on health and dispenser of medicines. It is perhaps time for the advisory drug-orientated role of the pharmacist to be more proactive than has recently been the case and to better complement the technically orientated role which has been dominant. Examples of some of the new roles proposed are a greater involvement in repeat prescribing (Audit Commission, 1994), and in the more extensive provision of over-the-counter (OTC) advice (DoH and Royal Pharmaceutical Society of Great Britain, 1992).

Self-medication is a cost-effective component of all health care systems, whether they are privately or publicly funded. The full potential of self care by patients has previously been limited because of legal restrictions on the range of drugs available for sale from pharmacies. However, there have been recent government-led moves, in many countries, to increase the number of such drugs, previously available only on prescription, by a re-regulation process which has been termed 'depomming' by the MCA. This has been supported by the pharmaceutical profession and the pharmaceutical industry. Although initially circumspect, the medical profession too seems to be coming to accept greater deregulation (Anon, 1992a; Spencer and Edwards, 1992; Erwin *et al.*, 1996). Total de-regulation (i.e. to general sales status) of some potent medicines, such as ibuprofen, is also being piloted (Anon, 1995a). This has raised more concerns amongst health care professionals.

International and UK re-regulation of drugs

The principals of re-regulation have also been supported by the World Health Organization (Levin, 1988). The conclusions of their report on self-medication in Europe were for 'a framework of orderly development, including reforms in professional education and practice'.

In 1989 Denmark was amongst the first of the northern European countries to re-regulate a large number of medicines, including cimetidine (Spencer and Edwards, 1992). Since then other European countries, for example Finland, have also rapidly increased the pace at which medicines are being reclassified. In the period January 1990 to December 1994, 50 products were switched including products such as hormone replacement therapies (HRT), haemorrhoid treatments, antihistamines, nicotine replacement therapies (NRTs), non-steroid anti-inflammatories (NSAIDs), and vaginal imidazoles were involved, a list with interesting similarities to the situation in the UK (*Financial Times*, 1994).

In contrast, changes have occurred much more slowly in some other countries, notably those previously in the Communist block. In Slovakia, for example, it is perceived that people need more education in self-medication before the regulations should be allowed to catch up with European Commission legislation. It seems surprising, therefore, that contraceptives and antidepressants feature in their list of expected OTC switches.

In the US, with their two classifications of 'prescription only' or 'general sale' medicines, there is ongoing debate about limiting the sale of selected non-prescription medications to pharmacies only. A study by Gore and Thomas (1995), based on a random postal survey of the general public, showed that stores with pharmacists provided better information to customers on selection and appropriate use of non-prescription medicines, and the authors argue that this provides support for the third category of drugs to be introduced in the US. In the meantime, even under their two-category system, more than 50 prescription drugs have been switched to non-prescription status in the past 20 years (Charupatanapong, 1994) and in general the spectrum of medicine available without a prescription is similar to that in the UK, including vaginal antifungal treatments. However, proposals to switch salbutamol and topical erythromycin have been blocked. In Australia salbutamol has been re-regulated but there have been concerns over the subsequent control of asthma and there are proposals to recategorize it as a POM (Gibson *et al.*, 1993).

The re-regulation process started slowly in the UK, with ibuprofen and loperamide (1983), terfenadine (1984), and hydrocortisone 1% cream (1985), but it has continued steadily with the support of the government (Bottomley, 1989), the Royal Pharmaceutical Society (DoH, 1992; Council of the Royal Pharmaceutical Society, 1995), and, to a limited extent, the Royal College of General Practitioners (Royal College of General Practitioners, 1995). A list of the recently re-regulated (or de-pommed) medicines in the UK is shown in Table 10.1.

Table 10.1 *A chronological list of medicines whose UK status has changed from POM to P[1] (1983–1996)*

Date	Ingredient	Date	Ingredient
1983	ibuprofen	1993	tioconazole (vaginal)
	loperamide	(cont.)	nicotine 4 mg gum
1984	terfenadine		hydrocortisone (oral pellet)
1985	hydrocortisone 1%		aluminium chloride
	(topical)		hexahydrate (topical)
1986	miconazole	1994	diclofenac (topical)
1988	ibuprofen sr and topical		felbinac (topical)
1989	astemizole		piroxicam (topical)
	mebendazole		flunisolide (nasal spray)
	dextromethorphan		ranitidine
1991	nicotine 2 mg gum		minoxidil (topical)
1992	hyoscine N butyl bromide		Adcortyl in Orabase
	nicotine patches		Anusol Plus HC ointment
	vaginal imidazoles		Anusol Plus HC
	hydrocortisone with		suppositories
	crotamiton (topical)	1995	hydroxyzine hydrochloride
	carbenoxolone		pyrantel embonate
	paracetamol and		fluconazole
	dihydrocodeine		ketoconazole (topical)
1993	loratidine		hydrocortisone (rectal)
	aciclovir (topical)		cadexomer iodine
	acrivastine		budesonide (nasal)
	cetirizine	1996	azelastine (nasal)
	ketoprofen (topical)		Nizatidine
	cimetidine		Hydrocortisone/lignocaine
	famotidine		perianal spray
	Beclomethasone		Mebeverine hydrochloride
	dipropionate (nasal)		Aciclovir
	Mebendazole (multiple dose)		Clotrimazole with
	Pseudoephedrine sr		hydrocortisone
	sodium cromoglycate (ophthalmic)		

[1] *Royal Pharmaceutical Society 1997 Prescription only medicines reclassified to pharmacy only medicines. Technical Information Department of the Royal Pharmaceutical Society of Great Britain: London.*

Future re-regulations are inevitable and various lists have been proposed, such as the much quoted 'list of 51' (Odd, 1992) or the more conservative one included in the consultative document *Pharmaceutical care: the future of community pharmacy* (DoH and Royal Pharmaceutical Society of Great Britain, 1992). This suggested that prescription controls could 'with advantage' be removed from a list of eight products. To date, of these eight, only a compound antibiotic ointment for the treatment of superficial bacterial skin infections and chloramphenicol 0.5% eye drops for eye infections remain POM. Other target preparations for future re-regulation include oral contraceptives and the 'morning after' pill (Lancet, 1993; Drife, 1993); this has the support of both the Royal College of General Practitioners (1995) and the General Medical Services Committee of the British Medical Association (1995). The most recent medicine to be proposed for re-regulation is a nasal application of budesonide (Anon, 1995b).

The consensus criteria for re-regulation are currently said to be that the drug should be of proven safety, of low toxicity in overdose, and for the treatment of minor 'self-limiting' conditions. The last of these is a vague definition which might already appear to be applied in a less stringent way than was originally envisaged, for example the availability of treatments for vaginal infections.

These criteria are applied now, but historically this has not always been the case; aspirin and paracetamol are widely used by the general public, but are not safe in overdose; glyceryl trinitrate tablets and oral theophylline are a further two examples of preparations which have long been available for P sale, although they could not be said to be for the treatment of self-limiting conditions and nor are they without side effects (Spencer and Edwards, 1992). Their P availability is, however, less widely known and the need for doctors to be more aware of this fact has been highlighted to avoid the potentially fatal combination of OTC and prescribed theophylline (Thomas, 1986). The rule of a self-limiting condition has not been applied rigorously in Australia where salbutamol inhalers were made available without a prescription in the early 1980s (Gibson *et al.*, 1993), though under current review. Their change in status was refused in the UK (A Wade, personal communication, 1991).

Although the current European position encourages re-regulation, it is still an expensive process. The application may be on a brand basis, for example Adcortyl in Orabase, or on an ingredient basis, for example for the vaginal imidazoles, and initiated by either a professional grouping (for example the Royal Pharmaceutical Society of Great Britain) or the industry.

If the initiative has come from the industry as opposed to the professional bodies, subsequent marketing will be used to optimize sales and ensure a viable product and an adequate return on investment. This includes direct advertising to the public, which can lead to problems in practice. The advertising is regulated by the industry under the auspices of the Proprietary Association of Great Britain, and standards have recently been raised to come into line with the 1992 European Pharmaceutical Advertising Directive (Proprietary Association of Great Britain, 1994).

Finally, although the net move is towards the re-regulation of medicines from POM to P, the status of all medicines is constantly under revision Europe-wide (Levin, 1988). There was an outcry from the pharmaceutical profession (Stroh,

1995) when small packs of ibuprofen 200 mg (12s) were further reclassified from P to GSL status (Anon, 1995a). This is de-regulation, as all restrictions on the sale are then removed. Conversely it was announced within a week that carbaryl, a treatment for headlice, would be restricted from P to POM because of evidence of possible carcinogenicity (Anon, 1995b).

Economic considerations to re-regulation

The DoH (1994) has suggested that £45 million could be saved if the numbers of prescriptions for preparations of medicines of limited clinical value were reduced. Many of these are available OTC.

In the UK, sales of OTC drugs have been increasing by 8% per annum since the mid 1980s. However, there has been no change in the average number of GP consultations, which have remained relatively constant at approximately four per person per year since 1979. (Chaplin, 1993; McCormick *et al.*, 1995.) Are the public simply consuming more drugs, as has happened in America (Eng and McCormick, 1990), rather than substituting the pharmacist for the GP as might perhaps have been hoped for?

OTC purchase of drugs can save patients' money as well as time and opportunity costs. Patients are saved the costs of visiting the physician followed by a subsequent visit to the pharmacist (although for non-employed patients who walk to clinics such costs are minimal). For those patients who would normally pay a prescription charge the savings will be dependent on the price of the reregulated product. There are already many prescription specialities which are cheaper than the current prescription charge if bought directly. A recent *Drug and Therapeutics Bulletin* lists these (1995). The picture is different if the patient is normally exempt from the prescription charge, and the only savings then are the indirect non-drug costs. If costs are defined to include both monetary and non-monetary elements, it has been shown that the over-the-counter availability of topical 1% hydrocortisone saved patients in the UK £2 million in 1987 alone (Ryan and Yule, 1990).

Savings may also be made by the NHS as drugs become available OTC. The government incurs two main costs in the prescribing of a drug; the costs of the physician's time, and the cost of the drug and the payment for its dispensing, whether it be by pharmacist or dispensing doctor. NHS indirect savings from the depomming of loperamide were estimated to be £0.13 million in 1985, £0.15 million in 1986, and £0.32 million in 1987 (Ryan and Yule 1990). Use of standard economic models of supply and demand can also be shown to demonstrate the economic advantages of switching (Ryan and Bond, 1994).

The theoretical savings from POM to P switches may not all be realized for a variety of reasons, one of which could be that currently 83% of prescriptions and 60% of patients do not incur the prescription levy (Jones, 1994; Prescription Pricing Authority, 1994). Thus the incentive to actually buy an OTC medicine may be countered by financial implications.

Further encouragement for the potential savings are that with the introduction of fundholding, GPs may be more likely to keep prescribing costs down by encouraging OTC purchase and self-medication wherever possible. It is already common practice for pharmacists to advise patients if the product prescribed by the GP is cheaper to buy OTC, the two professions working together to reduce prescribing costs.

Dunnell has suggested (1973) a change not only in the threshold at which illness is seen as justifying sickness absence, but also in the levels at which medicine taking is appropriate. This is based on evidence at that time, which indicated that the number of spells of certified sickness absence had increased, that less serious illness was increasingly regarded as justification for absence from work, that there was an increased consumption of prescribed and non-prescribed medicines, but that there was no evidence of an increase in the number of GP consultations. One of the perceived and anticipated advantages of changing the POM status of medicines would be to shift some of the cost of health care provision from the public to the private sector; will it merely change the patterns of drug consumption, or increase total consumption? It is as yet too early to predict the global effects of the changes, although there are indications of two possible scenarios, depending on whether the drug treatment is for an acute or a longer term condition.

Drugs used for the treatment of minor, acute self-limiting disease may indeed be expected largely to disappear from prescribing statistics. An example of this sort of drug would be topical aciclovir (Zovirax) used in the treatment of herpes labialis (cold sores). Inspection of SPA data shows that this has occurred (personal communication, F. Hickey, 1994) and potential UK savings of £900 000 have been identified, see Fig. 10.1.

However, a possibly more complex picture could evolve with drugs such as the H_2 blockers. These drugs are generally marketed at a lower dose than their

Fig. 10.1 *Number of prescriptions for aciclovir (Zovirax) 5% cream. Data from quarterly SPA level 2 data (section 13.10) for Grampian Health Board*

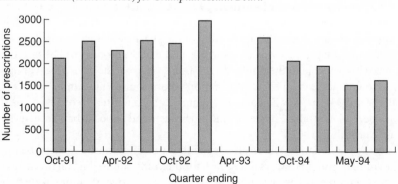

POM counterparts (raising concerns about efficacy), and can be used to treat long-term symptoms which may be associated with serious disease. Oster *et al.*, (1990) predicted for the US that if the H_2 antagonists were switched to OTC status, there would be an increase of people self-medicating for dyspepsia from 61.8% (of all indigestion sufferers) to 64.1%, that people seeking medical advice would drop by 1 108 000 per year, and that 1200 cases of gastric cancer would self-medicate before seeking medical advice, although the median time from onset to medical advice would not change.

Purchase of H_2 blockers to treat transient dyspepsia will result in a shift of the drug distribution mechanism from general medical practice to the community pharmacist and the public. The longer term implications could mean a greater volume of prescribed H_2 blockers as the public learn of the existence of an effective treatment yet are not prepared to pay long-term for it (and nor should the community pharmacist allow long-term use if supervising the sales in accordance with the P licence). Secondly, the fact that less effective doses are being purchased may mean that the GP, faced with a patient who has received no benefit from a H_2 blocker (the first line treatment), may go straight to the second line more expensive prescription (such as a proton pump inhibitor), not because he or she is unaware of the difference, but because of the overall balance of odds and a time-saving strategy. This is confirmed by prescribing statistics which indicate that the prescribing of H_2 antagonists has levelled off but, if the proton pump inhibitors are included, the antiulcer drug market continues to rise.

Finally, the industry has been suffering as a result of the moves to curb NHS spending on drugs. Evidence from the US would indicate that the commercial benefit of switching is very great (Macarthur, 1993). Thus the industry is looking to the OTC market to extend the brand life of existing prescription products which they can advertise to the public, yet continue to receive reimbursement for NHS prescriptions (Hardisty, 1990).

Legislation for non-prescription drugs

Every country other than the US has more than one legal category for non-prescription medicines (Macarthur, 1992) and switches normally occur to the next most restrictive category after POM. This normally implies that sale will be from a pharmacy under the supervision of the pharmacist, that counselling will be provided on product selection and use, and that the product will be stored in a place inaccessible to the public. In Australia, pharmacists have a legal obligation to give advice and elicit information before some drugs can be sold OTC (Barber, 1993). In New Zealand, it is required that a written record be made of the sale, and Australia, France, Spain, and Switzerland impose a ban on advertising (Macarthur, 1992).

In the Netherlands, where all self-medication drugs must be placed behind the counter, patients always have to ask for them and counselling on the drugs is reported more frequently than in Sweden where the drugs are more likely to be self selected (Blom *et al.*, 1993). Barber (1993) has recommended that all drugs that change from POM to P status should be sold in person by the pharmacist for the first 3 years. This sort of restriction could be imposed legally or at the professional discretion of the pharmacist. The new supervision protocols imposed by the Royal Pharmaceutical Society in Great Britain (from January 1995), puts in place a mechanism for the latter approach.

Since the philosophy behind re-regulation is based on the treatment of self-limiting disease there may sometimes be examples of switched products which could be used both for the treatment of self-limiting disease and also for longer term non-self-limiting conditions. The regulations may therefore be used to restrict the use of such a drug to an appropriate indication, or only after professional judgment. This practice has been formalized by the consensus development of clinical community pharmacy guidelines (Bond and Grimshaw, 1995).

Just as drugs can be reclassified, the legislation also allows for a change of indication. For example, topical hydrocortisone was originally deregulated only for allergic dermatitis but the restrictions were relaxed in a second generation switch so that it is now also allowed to be sold for eczema (although the original restriction regarding use on the face and genital areas remains). This move has partially addressed the confusion as to the indications for sale of the product, but raises the issue of whether restrictive symptoms for OTC use should be by legislation or professional consensus.

Liability issues and risks

The liability of community pharmacists when prescribing P medicines is complex. The manufacturer is liable should the patient suffer an untoward event attributable to the medicine. This assumes that the drug has been sold in an original container or that, in accordance with good professional practice, the pharmacist has identified the manufacturer and lot number on any repackaged product. However, the community pharmacist may be liable if it can be proved that his or her professional judgment in selling the medicine was in error (R. Rogers, personal communication, 1994). Furthermore, he or she has the responsibility to ensure that the product sale complies with any restrictive regulations. All community pharmacists are required by their Code of Ethics to have an indemnity policy, and the statutory committee of the Royal Pharmaceutical Society fulfils a disciplinary role (Appelbe and Harrison, 1993). In addition, complaints can be made to the Health Authorities in England and Wales, although to date these are relatively rare and the vast majority relate to prescribed medicines (Smith and Weidner, 1994).

Pharmacist malpractice law is case-made rather than statute-based. Americans are well known for being a 'litiginous group of people' (Brushwood, 1995), and in the US a new trend has established increased expectations of pharmacists, who are expected to prevent harm from drug therapy, in addition to fulfilling their long established responsibility to accurately dispense a medical doctor's prescription. This trend is set in the context of the expanded role of the pharmacist and concomitant further professional expectations. Although Brushwood does not quote examples from non-prescribed medicines, it would seem logical to extend the analogy of 'preventing harm from drug therapy' in this context in both the US and the UK.

The benefits of re-regulation have been discussed, but what are the risks? The potential for established OTC drugs to cause serious adverse drug reactions or significant interaction is well documented (Po, 1990). These are most likely to occur in the elderly, because of age-related pharmacodynamic and pharmacokinetic changes, and also because of problems such as difficulties in reading labels, anxiety, disability, poorer health, and multiple drug use (Rantucci and Segal, 1991). Patients on prescription medicines in Australia have been shown to use as many OTC products as the rest of the population, with 15% causing a theoretical risk of interaction with prescribed medications (Chua *et al.*, 1991). The further potential for risks arising from re-regulation is twofold; more potent medicines are available for OTC sale and are therefore used more widely, and there is a lack of physician intervention in a serious disease.

Post-marketing surveillance and phase IV studies of newly licensed drugs already identify problems which have not been identified in the selected populations used for the phase III clinical trials providing evidence for licensing applications (see Chapter 4). By analogy, the wider use of some previously POMs in wider patient groupings may well expose further, previously unknown, problems or side effects (Barber, 1993). The relevance of this can be illustrated by problems arising with astemizole and terfenadine after 'switching', namely the risk of ventricular arrhythmias at high doses (CSM, 1992). There were also two fatalities in 1987 from bronchospasm after a single dose of ibuprofen bought OTC (CSM, 1987), and there are reports of asthma induced by topical NSAIDs. Indeed 18% of drug-induced illness leading to hospital admission was shown to be due to OTC drugs (Caranas *et al.*, 1974), even before the recent wave of switches.

The lack of physician intervention in a serious disease is also a major concern, as treatment of symptoms may lead to the masking of more serious conditions for which early medical intervention is appropriate (DoH and Royal Pharmaceutical Society of Great Britain, 1992). The example already presented is the use of OTC H_2 blockers to treat symptoms perceived to be related to dyspepsia which could result in the masking of symptoms caused by gastric carcinoma. Similarly, the launch of OTC treatments for candidiasis could result in failure to identify bacterial vaginosis and sexually transmitted diseases. Mild attacks of genital herpes and psychosexual problems have also been listed as causing symptoms which could mimic vaginal thrush (Mitchell and Bradbeer, 1992).

Herxheimer *et al.* (1993) have recommended that pharmacists only recommend drugs from a list of nationally agreed medicines. Such a list should possibly be used as a basis for each community pharmacist constructing their own formulary, as has also been proposed by Noyce (1992). In so doing, they should follow all the agreed guidelines for general practice formulary construction

(Grant *et al.*, 1985) thus enabling them to objectively select a limited number of treatments in each therapeutic category for which they would be familiar with costs, side effects, and contraindications. This could increase the recently reported low impact of clinical factors (4%) and equivalently decrease the influence of advertising as influences on a community pharmacist's prescribing decision (Emmerton *et al.*, 1994). The importance of commercial advertising influences, which that study demonstrated, reflects a similar situation in medical decision making (Taylor and Bond, 1991).

The jointly agreed written supervision protocols now required under the professional Code of Ethics of the Royal Pharmaceutical Society of Great Britain will be an aid to ensuring that sales are made appropriately, to explicitly define the supervision requirement, and to obviate previous interpretations of the supervision requirement sometimes fulfilled by an apparently token bell-ringing. This, together with the new formal training requirements for all counter staff involved in the sale of medicines (Evans and Moclair, 1994), should reduce the risks of inappropriate sale.

Are any risks from OTC medication perceived by the patients? The study of counselling previously reported (Rantucci and Segal, 1986) showed that even with knowledge, patients still acted irresponsibly and dangerously, as evidenced by the concurrent consumption of alcohol and antihistamines. Another US study (Charupatanapong, 1994) showed that better educated, middle-aged females were more likely to perceive risk with OTC use of medication than were younger, less educated, male clients. The implications are that pharmacists should be encouraged to consciously direct more counselling to their younger male customers.

The hard sell approach by the industry, with intensive advertising campaigns, could reduce patient perceptions of the possible risks associated with a product, for example therapeutically reducing cimetidine to simple antacid level. By failing to reinforce the need for consultation with the pharmacist about the suitability of the product, and consideration of alternative treatments, they promote a philosophy of the right to a 'pill for every ill' with its inherent benefits and risks.

Physicians and OTC recommendation: implications for practice

There are two main ways in which the use of OTC medications will affect general practice consultations. Firstly there is evidence (Williams *et al.*, 1996) that problems can arise as a result of interactions between prescription and non-prescription medicines. Are questions about prior and continuing self-medication asked often enough, particularly in the elderly who are often on polypharmacy regimes? Often several prescription drugs and OTC purchases may be within the same therapeutic group, for example laxatives or analgesics. Presenting symptoms may be the result of inappropriate and unknown prior self-medication (for example constipation resulting from excessive use of codeine-containing analgesics). Important symptoms may be masked because of prior self-medication. If re-regulation continues these reported incidents may become more frequent.

Secondly, should GPs be advising patients to purchase their medicines OTC if the preparation is available? This could have tangible economic benefits for the fundholding GP, and reduce the prescribing budgets for those in the Indicative Prescribing Scheme (IPS). A recent government statement has indicated that this would not be in contravention of the terms and conditions of service of GPs (Kelly, 1994). The GP is left in a position of either deciding that patients should bear the increased cost personally or making decisions as to who should receive the benefit of free healthcare.

Factors supporting wider self-medication and OTCs

General practitioners should be reassured that the drugs which are depommed are considered to be safe, as a wide range of experts have considered extensive evidence before switching a drug. There is also the increasing belief that patients should be encouraged to be more responsible for their own health and that doctors should assist patient self-reliance and self-management. By encouraging the wider uptake of OTC medication, patients will be empowered and will possibly reduce their costs.

Patients should use their community pharmacist more, not just after a recommendation to purchase a drug but also possibly on future occasions for advice prior to a visit to the surgery. Just as a large part of general practice workload may, when appropriate, be devolved to (often nursing-related) members of the primary health care team, some care should also be devolved to the community pharmacist.

Allowing the pharmacist to have more drugs available could be of particular advantage to patients. Community pharmacists are said to be the most accessible of all health care professionals as their premises are located in local high streets and open all day. Drugs necessary for immediate use, such as contraceptives (Lancet, 1993) and postcoital contraception (Drife, 1993), or those whose prescription is limited by regulation such as the 'blacklist' could be readily obtained if depommed as proposed.

Factors mitigating against wider re-regulation

Despite these advantages of OTCs, there are at least as many disadvantages. Although it is not uncommon for patients to consult their doctor when self-medication (which does not necessarily imply even an OTC purchase but merely time) would have likely been effective, these contacts should not be viewed negatively. Such consultations offer time for opportunistic health promotion, counselling about other long-term medication, and updating on other pre-existing conditions.

The risks of some reregulated products theoretically masking more serious symptoms has been discussed. Wider use of more potent OTC medications could also result in a higher incidence of interactions between prescription and non-prescription specialities. For example, the recently reregulated cimetidine has the potential to change the pharmacokinetics of other drugs such as warfarin, phenytoin, or theophylline which are metabolized by the cytochrome P450 pathway, and causes documented confusional problems in the elderly. Although pharmacy guidelines for the use of cimetidine specifically exclude the elderly (Bond, 1994), the wider availability of the drug will inevitably mean that there is a greater chance of these problems occurring.

The wider availability of more drugs may also tend to encourage the 'pill for every ill' mentality. At a time when there is an increased awareness that a prescription is not always the best treatment, when we are trying to discourage patients' dependence on benzodiazepines and hypnotics, should we be supporting increased self-medication with OTCs? The necessity for drug companies to recoup their investment in re-regulation by advertising direct to the public could create inappropriate demand for a drug. A pharmacist should be able to monitor this, but not necessarily the pharmacy assistant who may transact the sale. The counter-argument that all drugs which are re-regulated should be safe, even if used wrongly, is clearly flawed thinking. Furthermore, many of the recent re-regulations are in America where, since there is no P category, the supervision of the pharmacist is not legally required.

It has been argued that pharmacists, operating from commercial premises will be under pressure to make a sale of an OTC product so that the profit will in effect provide a fee for the consultation. The remuneration package for community pharmacy is currently being restructured. Until recently the global sum for the pharmaceutical service was allocated on the basis of numbers of prescriptions dispensed. At that time the dispensing fee per item provided a greater profit than the profit on the sale of an OTC, so it was in the pharmacist's interest, if in doubt, to refer a patient to the doctor. The new mechanism for remuneration has topsliced a small amount from the global sum to be paid to pharmacists as a professional fee which will reimburse in part OTC counselling and obviate the need for this to come from a commercial sale. Community pharmacists remain professionals who should, and no doubt for the most part do, put the needs of their patients before commercial profit. There are many situations where doctors are also open to similar temptations of personal gain if they did not act in an altruistic and professional way.

A final factor against the wider availability of OTCs might be a paradoxical increase in prescribing costs. Patients with experience of an effective but expensive drug off prescription may demand the drug on prescription. To date there is no evidence for this consequence, but it must remain a theoretical possibility which future re-regulations might encourage.

Recommendations for the future

Issues surrounding re-regulation can no longer be ignored by clinicians (Bradley and Bond, 1995). The benefits and the problems associated with depomming need to be addressed by recommendations under four broad headings: issues for general practice, issues for the patient, issues for the pharmacist and finally and most importantly issues to be addressed jointly by GPs and community pharmacists.

For general practice, it should become routine to seek information from the patient on prior self-medication both for the presenting symptom and for concurrent symptoms. Furthermore this information should be recorded in the patient's records (both written notes and computerized). Computerized systems used for detecting prescribed drug interactions also need to be programmed to include OTCs. This applies not only to newer OTCs but also all established preparations. Additionally the GP's 'social' policy on who should buy their own drugs and who should get a free prescription should also be discussed, clarified, and made consistent at least between partners. The final decision on this will have to be a personal one.

Patients must be better educated to consider when their conditions need medical help and when advice from the community pharmacist could be equally efficacious. It must also be made clear to them that they have a choice under these circumstances, and that the GP is still there to treat them should they so wish. Patients should better understand that sometimes there is no need to take any drug and that time alone will result in recovery, although palliative treatment might make the interim easier. They should also realize that simply because they have been able to buy their medicine without a prescription this in no way implies that this medication should not be treated with respect. If a patient is asked what other medicine is being taken they must understand that OTCs are items that doctors need to know about.

Similarly, pharmacists should also check concomitant medication when selling OTC preparations, particularly when prescribing the newer, more potent OTCs over the counter. This can be done by questioning the patient, as is done routinely, but also by consulting the computerized medication records which pharmacies now hold for most regular patients. To date the primary use of these has been for dispensary checks and labelling, but the opportunity exists for the systems to be put to better use; records of the sale of selected OTCs should almost certainly be recorded alongside the records of dispensed medication.

Finally we shall consider the general practice–community pharmacy interface. Most pharmacists are very aware of their professional responsibilities towards their patients and in general err on the side of caution when advising patients. In other words, they would be more likely to refer a patient to the GP than otherwise. There is professional concern that the newly deregulated products should be used appropriately (Scottish Department Executive, 1992) and launches of new products would now appear to be routinely accompanied by training articles and *aides memoires* in the professional journals, and also increasingly sophisticated training packages from the industry.

A better way might be a method piloted for the newly deregulated cimetidine (Bond and Grimshaw, 1995). A multidisciplinary group including a gastro-enterologist, GPs, and community pharmacists together developed an algorithmic guideline for the treatment of dyspepsia, including use of standard antacids, H_2 blockers, and referral to general practice. This has been well received by local community pharmacists and their associated GPs. This initiative not only resulted in guidelines which were acceptable to both professions and the hospital specialist, but also allowed a better mutual understanding of the *modus operandi* of both professions so that the community pharmacists understood better the concerns expressed by their medical colleagues, and the doctors better understood the abilities and training of the pharmacists and were reassured of their ability to safely advise their patients.

Under the current UK climate of internal markets and patient responsibility, and world-wide attitudes to self-medication, it is likely that re-regulation will continue. On balance there are many advantages for patient, physician, and healthcare systems (Hobbs, 1994), in addition to providing an opportunity for a more integrated primary health care role for the community pharmacist. If the precautions discussed are adopted, then all interested groups will reap the benefits of the changes whilst minimizing the possible adverse consequences.

References

Anon, (1992). Royal College of GPs accepts pharmacy report with reservations. *Pharmaceutical Journal*, **249**, 305.

Anon, (1995a). GSL ibuprofen product to be marketed this month. *Pharmaceutical Journal*, **254**, 12.

Anon, (1995b). POM-to-P shift proposed for budesonide and P-to-POM for carbaryl. *Pharmaceutical Journal*, **255**, 138.

Appelbe, G. E., Harrison, I. (1993). The statutory committee and convictions. *Pharmaceutical Journal*, **251**, 565–7.

Audit Commission (1994). *A prescription for improvement*. HMSO, London.

Baker, M. (1993). *POM to P: who controls? Proceedings of members' meeting July 1993*. Proprietary Association of Great Britain, London.

Barber, N. (1993). Drugs: from prescription only to pharmacy only. *British Medical Journal*, **307**, 640.

Blom, A. Th. G., Kam, A. L., Bakker, A. (1993). Patient counselling in community pharmacy. *Journal of Social and Administrative Pharmacy*, **10**(2), 53–62.

Bond, C. M. (1994). Clinical guidelines for the treatment of dyspepsia in community pharmacies. *Pharmaceutical Journal*, **25**, 228–9.

Bond, C. M., Grimshaw, J. M. (1995). Multidisciplinary guideline development: a case study from community pharmacy. *Health Bulletin*, **53**(1), 26–33.

Bottomley, V. (1989). *Reported in* POM to P call to meet government's health challenge. *Pharmaceutical Journal*, **243**, 728.

Bradley, C. P., Bond, C. (1995). Increasing the number of drugs available over the counter: arguments for and against. *British Journal of General Practice*, **45**, 553–6.

Brushwood, D. B. (1995). The pharmacist's expanding legal responsibility for patient care. *Journal of Social and Administrative Pharmacy*, **12**(2), 53–62.

Caranas, G. J., Stewart, R. B., Clutt, L. E. (1974). Drug induced illness leading to hospitalisation. *Journal of the American Medical Association*, **228**, 713.

Chaplin, S. (1993). Sparse facts back the switch to OTC therapy. *MIMS Magazine* 12 October, 30–31.

Charupatanapong, N. (1994). Perceived likelihood of risks in self medication practices. *Journal of Social and Administrative Pharmacy*, **11**(1), 18–27.

Council of the Royal Pharmaceutical Society of Great Britain (1995). *Annual Report*. Pharmaceutical Press, London.

Chua, S., Benrimoj, S., Stewart, K. (1991). Usage of non-prescription medicines by hypertensive patients. *Journal of Social and Administrative Pharmacy*, **8**(1), 33–45.

Committee for Safety of Medicines and Medicines Control Agency (1987). Non-steroidal anti-inflammatory drugs (NSAIDs and asthma). *Current Problems in Pharmacovigilance*, **20**.

Committee for Safety of Medicines and Medicines Control Agency (1992). Astemizole and terfenadine *Current problems in Pharmacovigilance*, **35**.

DoH (1987). *Promoting better health*. Government White Paper, CM249, HMSO, London.

DoH (1989). *Secretaries of State for Health, Wales, Northern Ireland, and Scotland: Indicative prescribing budgets for general medical practitioners. (working paper 4)*. HMSO, London.

DoH (1992). *Statistical Bulletin*, **4**(4).

DoH (1994). EL (94) 2. See *Pharmaceutical Journal*, **252**, 211; **252**, 348.

DoH and Royal Pharmaceutical Society of Great Britain (1992). *Pharmaceutical care: the future for community pharmacy*. Royal Pharmaceutical Society, London.

Drife, J. O. (1993). Deregulating emergency contraception. *British Medical Journal*, **307**, 695–6.

Drug and Therapeutics Bulletin (1993). Medicines cheaper over the counter. *Drug and Therapeutics Bulletin*, **31**(15), suppl.

Dunnell, K. (1973). Medicine takers and hoarders. *Journal of the Royal College of General Practitioners*, **23**, Suppl. 2, 2–9.

Eng, H. J., McCormick, W. C. (1990). Assessment of the Florida pharmacist self-care consultant law using patient profile and prescription audit methods. *Drug Intelligence and Clinical Pharmacy Annals of Pharmacotherapy*, **24**, 931–4.

Emmerton, L., Gow, D. J., Berrimoj, S. I. (1994). Dimensions of pharmacists preferences for cough and cold products. *International Journal of Pharmeutical Practice*, 3, 27–32.

Erwin, J., Britten, N., Jones, R. (1996). General practitioners' views on over the counter sales by community pharmacists. *British Medical Journal*, **312**, 617–8.

European Community (1992). *Directive for medicines classification*. 92/26/EEC.

Evans, D., Moclair, A., (1994). Vocational qualifications for pharmacy support staff. *Pharmaceutical Journal*, **252**, 631.

Financial Times (1994). Finland steps up pace of switching. *OTC Business News* November 9–13.

General Medical Services Committee (1995) *reported in* More support for OTC emergency contraception. *Pharmaceutical Journal*, **254**, 572.

Gibson, P., Henry, D., Francis, L., Cruickshank, D., Dupen, F., Higginbotham, N., Henry, R., Sutherland, D. (1993). Association between availability of non prescription beta 2 agonist inhalers and under treatment of asthma. *British Medical Journal*, **306**, 1514–18.

Gore, M. R., Thomas, J. (1995). Non-prescription information services in pharmacies and alternative stores: implications for a third class of drugs. *Journal of Soc. and Admin. Pharm.*, **12**(2), 86–99.

Grant, G. B., Gregory, D. A., van Zwanenburg, T. D. (1985). Development of a limited formulary for general practice. *Lancet*, **327**, 1030–2.

Hardisty, B. (1990). The enigma of OTC advertising. *Pharmaceutical Journal*, **245**, 321.

Health Committee (1994). *Priority setting in the NHS: the NHS drugs budget*. HMSO, London.

Herxheimer, A., Upton, D., Spivey, P., Sharpe, D., Tugwell, C., Barrett, C. (1993). Wanted: a formulary for self care. *Pharmaceutical Journal*, **251**, 179.

Hobbs, F. D. R. (1994). Community pharmacy links to general practice. *15th Unichem Annual Conference, Vancouver, Canada*. Unichem.

Jones, P. (1994). *POM to P: pharmaceutical implications*. Lothian Health Board, Edinburgh.

Kelly, S. (1994). Minister supports GPs in recommending OTCs. In *OTC Directory 1994/1995*. Proprietary Association of Great Britain, London.

Lancet, (1993). Editorial. OCs o-t-c? *Lancet*, **342**, 565–6.

Levin, L. S. (1988). Self medication in Europe: some perspectives on the role of the pharmacist. In (1988) *The role and function of the pharmacist in Europe. Report of a WHO working group*, ed. I. Lund and G. Dukes. Styx Publications, Groningen.

Macarthur, D. (1992). *Pharmaceutical pricing in Japan.* Donald Macarthur, Dorking.

Macarthur, D. (1993). *OTC switches—hope or hype?* Donald Macarthur, Dorking.

McCormick, A., Fleming, D., Charlton, J. (1995). *Morbidity statistics from general practice. Fourth national study 1991–2.* Office of Population Censuses and Surveys, Series MB5 No 3. HMSO, London.

Medicines Control Agency (1992). *Changing the legal classification of a prescription only medicine for human use.* MAL 77, MCA, London.

Mitchell, S., Bradbeer, C. (1992). Over-the-counter treatment for candidiasis: an opportunity to educate. *British Medical Journal,* **304**, 1648.

National Audit Office (1992). *Community Pharmacies in England.* HMSO, London.

Noyce, P. (1992). Rationalising the pharmacist's role. *International Journal of Pharm. Prac.,* **1**(3), 122–3.

Nuffield Foundation Committee of Enquiry (1986). *Pharmacy: a report to the Nuffield Foundation.* Nuffield Foundation: London.

Odd, R. (1992). *Proceedings of Medicines Control Agency POM to P seminar.* Royal Pharmaceutical Society of Great Britain, London.

Oster, G., Huse, D. M., Delea, T. E., Colditz, G. A., Richter, J. M. (1990). The risks and benefits of an Rx-to-OTC switch: the case of over-the-counter H2 blockers. *Medical Care,* **28**, 834–52.

Po, A. L. W. (1990). *Non-prescription drugs,* 2nd edn. Blackwell Scientific Publications, Oxford.

Prescription Pricing Authority (1994). *Annual Report.* PPA, Newcastle upon Tyne.

Proprietary Association of Great Britain (1994). *Code of standards of advertising practice for over-the-counter medicines.* PAGB, London.

Rantucci, M., and Segal, H. (1991). Hazardous non-prescription analgesic use by the elderly. *Journal of Social and Administrative Policy,* **3**(3), 81–91.

Royal College of General Practitioners (1993). Comment by the Royal College of General Practitioners on the Report of the Joint Working Party on the future role of the Community Pharmaceutical Services. In *1993 Members' Reference Book,* pp. 145–9. RCGP, London.

Royal College of General Practitioners (1995). *reported in* RCGP votes for emergency contraception OTC. *Pharmaceutical Journal,* **254**, 185.

Ryan, M., Yule, B. (1990). Switching drugs from prescription-only to over-the-counter availability: economic benefits in the United Kingdom. *Health Policy,* **16**, 233–9.

Ryan, M., Bond, C. (1994). Dispensing physician and prescribing pharmacists. *Pharmacoeconomics,* **5**(1), 8–17.

Scottish Department Executive (1992). Report on the council meeting of the Royal Pharmaceutical Society. *Pharmaceutical Journal*, **248**, 219.

Smith, F. J., Weidner, D. (1994). Complaints to family health services authorities about pharmacy services *International Journal of Pharm.Prac.*, **2**, 199–204.

Spencer, J., Edwards, C. (1992). Pharmacy beyond the dispensary: general practitioners' views. *British Medical Journal*, **304**, 1670–2.

Stroh, B. (1995). Medicines classification. *Pharmaceutical Journal*, **255**, 167.

Taylor, R. J., Bond, C. M. (1991). Change in the established prescribing habits of general practitioners: an analysis of first prescriptions in general practice. *British Journal of General Practice*, **41**, 244–8.

Thomas, C. E. (1986). Over-the-counter theophyllines. *Journal of the Royal College of General Practitioners*, **36**, 180.

Taylor, R. J., Bond, C. M. (1985). Limited list: limited effects? *British Medical Journal*, **291**, 518–20.

Williams, A., Clarke, G., Bond, C., Winfield, A., Ellerby, D. (1996). Domiciliary pharmaceutical care for older people—a feasibility study. *Pharmaceutical Journal*, **256**, 236–8.

CHAPTER ELEVEN

Prescribing a complementary therapy: an introduction to homoeopathy

Sheila Greenfield, Andy Wearn, and Mollie Hunton

Homoeopathy is one of an increasing number of therapeutic approaches to health problems that are proving more popular with patients and some doctors. These therapeutic approaches are sometimes referred to as 'alternative therapies' but this depiction of them is too antagonistic and rejecting by allopathic medicine based on scientific rationalism. A preferable term is 'complementary therapies', which suggest their use alongside allopathic medicine. This term accords such therapies their proper role, as it does not seek to deny patient access to modern medicine and yet acknowledges that modern medicine does have its limitations and complementary therapies can offer something beyond what may be achieved with conventional treatments alone.

There are a host of such complementary therapies, but homoeopathy is the only one that is completely appropriate to discuss in a book on prescribing. It is a complementary therapy prescribed in a manner similar to that used for the prescription of more conventional medicines. It is also prescribable on the NHS; indeed, homoeopathy enjoys a special place among complementary therapies as it is the only one that has been available on the NHS since its inception.

This chapter will define homoeopathy, describe its origins and underlying principles, and refer to recent attempts to put the therapy on a sounder scientific footing through research. The chapter will also provide some examples of the use of homoeopathic remedies to give readers a flavour of how homoeopathy is used in a practical sense. For readers who are interested in pursuing this therapy further there is a list of suggested additional reading, although they are also strongly advised to seek specific training on this treatment method before embarking on using it on their own patients.

Definitions

Homoeopathy is a holistic therapeutic system of administering medicines after assessing the patient's constitution, symptoms, and signs of disease. The aim is to restore the inner balance of the patient. The founding father of homoeopathy, a German physician named Samuel Hahnemann (1755–1844), described this 'inner vital force' as the *dynamis* and suggested that an 'untuned' *dynamis* resulted in disease (Hahnemann, as translated by Kinzli *et al.*, 1983). Homoeopathic remedies would assist the body in restoring this balance. At the same time mainstream medicine was postulating that disease was caused by some undiscovered entity within the organism. Contemporary treatments largely involved purging, crude dosing with poisons, venesection, and basic surgery.

Hahnemann observed that medicines frequently produced new symptoms and signs in the patient. He postulated that prescribing medicines or substances which produced a certain pattern of symptoms and signs might be used to treat diseases with a similar profile (Hippocrates had made a similar observation in the 5th century BC, which had been largely forgotten). The symptoms or physiological effects produced by substances on healthy subjects, 'provers', were noted and the same substance was then used as a remedy to treat patients with similar symptoms caused by disease.

From the success of his experiments came the central principle of homoeopathy, *similia similibus curentur*; the principle that 'like cures like'. It is from this 'law of similars' that homoeopathy derives its name (*homoios*, like; *pathos*, suffering). Modern medicine is often referred to as allopathic (*allos*, other; *pathos*, suffering). Allopathic treatment is based on administering therapies which counteract symptoms, such as antibiotics, antihistamines, and antiemetics.

The remedies used in homoeopathy are all made from naturally occurring minerals, plants or their extracts and animal products. Many of these raw substances are known poisons, such as belladonna (deadly nightshade). Ingestion of the raw substance, which contains atropine, causes fever, flushing, headache, pupillary dilatation, and delirium. It is used principally for headache, fever, and inflammation, with specific use in cases of scarlet fever, acute tonsillitis, otitis media and glue ear, throbbing headaches, and sunstroke.

Remedies, termed *nosodes*, are made specifically from disease products or cultures. They are used in the acute phase of an illness, or some time afterwards if there are chronic sequelae. Remedies for allergy are made from the allergen, whether natural or synthetic.

Hahnemann's next step in developing homoeopathic treatments was to dilute the raw substance to a concentration where aggravation of or new symptoms was minimal and beneficial effects maximal. First of all a solution must be produced. Soluble raw material or extract is either dissolved in water and/or absolute alcohol to make a 1 molar solution (or tincture). Insoluble material is crushed and ground up with lactulose in a process called *trituration*. After this the triturated substance becomes soluble and is dissolved in alcohol. Next the solutions are serially diluted by a factor of 10 (designated 'x' or 'D' dilutions), 100 (designated 'c' dilutions), or 1000 (designated 'M' dilutions) with distilled water and alcohol.

These dilutions are called *potencies*. For example, a solution diluted 12 times by a factor of 100 is termed a 12c potency. However, a vital part of the process in imbuing the remedy with activity is called *succussion*. This involves striking the vessel containing the solution on a firm but yielding surface many times between each dilution. Traditionally the surface used was a thick leather bound book such as the family bible, and modern automated production uses machines which imitate this action. Dilutions that were not succussed were found to be inactive by Hahnemann.

Remedies are available in a variety of formulations; tablets, pilules, globules, granules, powders, ointments, creams, and tinctures.

Trends in homoeopathy

Homoeopathy was first brought to Britain in 1827 by a Scottish doctor called Frederick Quin who founded the British Homoeopathic Society in 1844. Although generally accepted within the NHS as a legitimate form of therapy, with its availability on NHS prescription, homoeopathy has never been part of undergraduate teaching and has frequently been opposed by mainstream doctors, usually on the grounds that its mode of action is not known. Instead it has tended to be practised by a few enthusiasts and their converts. Over the last 20 years the popularity of complementary therapies as a whole has grown steadily in the general population and within medicine (MORI, 1989; Murray and Shepherd, 1993). In part this parallels the fashion for a more 'natural' and holistic health system. Patients increasingly express concerns about potential side effects of pharmacological and invasive treatments. There is often a disenchantment with prevailing options. (Brewin, 1993)

Homoeopathy is one of the more popular complementary therapies practised by or recommended by GPs (Swayne, 1989). In Europe the extent to which homoeopathy is practised varies considerably. In France up to 40% of the population use homoeopathy, whereas it is rarely used in Denmark. In Germany it is now a compulsory part of undergraduate training. Recent EC directives concerning licensing of medicines caused controversy because homoeopathic remedies were to be exempt. Conventional practitioners also expressed unhappiness over labelling, arguing that remedies should not be referred to as 'medicines' and that no claims should be made on the containers for special indications (Abbott, 1992). There, therefore, continue to be differences of opinion regarding homoeopathy and the legitimacy of its place in medicine.

Research on homoeopathic remedies

The biggest stumbling block for most people is in understanding how high dilutions of a substance can cause an effect. One mole of a substance contains 6.02252×10^{23} atoms or molecules (Avogadro's number). Therefore any potency higher than a 12c is highly unlikely to contain even a single molecule of the original substance. In effect a dilution of 12c or greater is simply water or alcohol. The explanation for its activity is thought to be due to the energy imparted by succussion and the solvent's 'memory' of the solute in the form of altered polymer structure through the creation of solvation cages (Gibson and Gibson, 1987). Although it is known that water crystals can take up a variety of different polymerized forms, the proposed effect of a solute after its removal is still hypothetical.

Trials of homoeopathic remedies have taken several forms, and the published data have indicated positive, negative, and equivocal results. The academic consensus is that there is no consensus. Studies have either determined the effect of 'potencies' on healthy subjects (Walach, 1993), investigated responses *in vitro* (Davenas *et al.*, 1988; Maddox *et al.*, 1988) or examined the efficacy of potencies in disease. Efficacy studies usually include a control, placebo, or mainstream treatment. The rigour of the methodology in published studies varies considerably.

A meta-analysis of controlled trials of homoeopathy in the *British Medical Journal* illustrates this well and concludes that there is still insufficient evidence to draw a definitive conclusion regarding efficacy (Kleijnen *et al.*, 1991). Of the 105 trials, 81 showed positive results. Trials were scored according to the rigour of their method, with 80% achieving less than 55 marks out of 100. However, of those scoring more than 55 marks, 73% had positive results.

Of the two best trials which appear in this meta-analysis, a trial using 30c homoeopathic potency of grass pollens against placebo in the treatment of hay fever gave a positive result and a trial of two homoeopathic medicines against placebo and untreated controls in the recovery of ileus following bowel surgery yielded a negative result (Reilly *et al.*, 1986; GRECHO, 1989). Lately a number of editorials have appeared in academic journals calling for both good quality research and alternative research approaches more suited to the different philosophy and practice of complementary medicine (Smith, 1995; Ernst, 1994). Recently published papers have looked at the effect of homoeopathic medicines in childhood upper respiratory tract infection (Deklerk *et al.*, 1994) and in pain control after oral surgery (Lokken *et al.*, 1995). Both had negative results.

Homoeopathy in general practice

In general practice, homoepathy is used to treat a range of acute and chronic conditions including those for which there is no specific allopathic treatment, such as glandular fever. Often it is used when traditional medicines have not helped or have produced side effects.

Local pharmacists increasingly stock homoeopathic medicines. They are cheap to buy, have an indefinite shelf life, and take up very little space to store. The GP can then prescribe, either on an FP10 or privately, or advise the patient to buy over the counter. A 15G 6c potency costs about £3.20 for 125 tablets and 15G of 30c costs about £3.85 (1997 prices).

Initially most doctors begin by administering remedies for common acute conditions, using a *Materia Medica*. This is a book containing all the known effects of the medicines (*provings*), having been tested on healthy human volunteers, or from toxicology. The doctor then matches the symptoms of the patient to the *Materia Medica* and when a good match is obtained, prescribes that remedy. If the symptoms are complicated, then a *Repertory* is used. This is a book containing lists of symptoms with remedies which are known to be effective. Hahnemann produced the first *Materia Medica* in 1810, and Kent introduced his first *Repertory* around 1910. Appendix I lists examples of remedies used to treat acute everyday problems within the usual constraints of the general practice consultation.

The potencies (or strengths) of remedies commonly used are 6c, 30c, and 200c. These are generally considered low, medium, and high potencies. The 6c is available OTC. It is best to start with 30c and get to know how to use it in acute situations before going on to chronic prescribing and using the other potencies. The higher potencies (e.g. 200c, 1M, and 10M) are used when the symptoms are mainly from the *mental sphere*. Homoeopathy divides the body's 'energy field' into physical, mental, emotional, and spiritual spheres. The mental sphere relates to rational thought as well as intuitive and imaginative sides of thinking. Problems in this sphere might became apparent by a comment from a patient such as 'feeling unwell after visiting a particular place'. The low potencies are used when the patient has had a prolonged illness, is on many orthodox medications or when overstimulation with a higher potency might aggravate the condition.

When Hahnemann first tested his medicines in the 1c, 2c, and 3c potencies he discovered that a proportion of patients developed aggravation, that is they became worse before getting better. The aggravations were greatest with 1c and least with 6c, which is why this potency is commonly used. Aggravations do occur when the symptom remedy match is very good, but they are not usually a problem. They seem to occur mainly when the illness has an allergic basis (e.g. asthma and eczema) and with remedies which are being used to desensitize patients (e.g. house dust or cat dander). Caution is needed, but there are no recorded cases of death from this method in the homoeopathic literature.

Taking homoeopathic medicines is simple. They are all absorbed from the buccal mucosa. They should be sucked, chewed, or crushed between two spoons and the powder administered or dissolved in a little water and put in the mouth (ideal for infants). The remedy is taken before food or drink and there should be no residual strong flavours in the mouth as these are thought to block the absorption of the remedy. The patient is also advised not to drink coffee, as caffeine seems to stop the remedy from working. Touching the tablets denatures them, so they are usually tipped out of the bottle into the cap or a spoon and then placed into the mouth.

Taking a case history

The symptoms of the presenting illness and how they affect the patient (*modalities*) are recorded; for example, the patient may complain that his osteoarthritic knee is painful and stiff (*symptoms*), worse when he starts to move about and better if he keeps going (*modalities*). Modalities are specific to that patient's reactions to his or her illness, and in the example above would match the remedy *Rhus Tox* exactly.

The precipitating factors in an illness are most important in homoeopathy. It is recognized that people sometimes become ill through emotional factors such as shock, grief, or fear and this may lead to physical symptoms. Patients often say that they have never felt well since a particular severe or prolonged illness, e.g. glandular fever. In this case the glandular fever nosode would be used. A nosode in conjunction with the constitutional remedy can be effective in restoring the patient to health. Homoeopathic medicines are used to treat many chronic problems including asthma and eczema, arthritis, depression, endometriosis and myalgic encephalitis. Homoeopathic medicines are also used to counteract the side effects of allopathic drugs, for 'general constitutional support' and for 'mental improvement'.

In order to prescribe in this way (*constitutional* prescribing) the clinician needs to know more about the patient's persona and response to illness. For example, if you give someone a small dose of pure arsenic they develop diarrhoea, vomiting, and weakness. After further doses other symptoms appear; icy coldness, restlessness, anxiety, and fears. The poison first affects the physical sphere and then the mental. In taking a case history for a chronic case the physical symptoms with their modalities are very important, but the mentals are considered the most important because they define the individual's reaction to their disease. Case histories are presented in Appendix II.

There are a number of conditions and situations for which there are no specific homoeopathic treatments. These include hypertension, contraception, and substitutes for insulin, thyroxine, vitamin B_{12}, and other hormone or replacement therapies.

It is obviously more difficult to prescribe a constitutional medicine in a 5 minute consultation, but some of the remedies are easy to pick out just by asking a few key questions, especially in children. With a difficult problem such as myalgic encephalitis a longer consultation or a few short consultations are necessary, as the case history will need to include the presenting symptoms with modalities, precipitating factors, the past and family histories, the general symptoms and the psychological profile. This takes time but gives good results.

Training and resources

Introductory courses, usually one whole day, are held in all UK health regions. These enable the doctor to acquire enough knowledge to make a start at homoeopathic prescribing. The Royal London Homoeopathic Hospital in Great Ormond Street, Glasgow Homoeopathic Hospital, Bristol Homoeopathic Hospital, and Oxford Homoeopathic Physicians Teaching group all run modular courses leading to the diploma in homoeopathy or to membership of the Faculty (MFHom). Fellows are elected by thesis or publication.

Tutorials are held regularly in Birmingham, Liverpool, Tunbridge Wells, and Manchester and in some of the regions of Scotland and the South West. Special courses are also held by the Pharmacy Dean to train pharmacists. Consultant physicians are available for out-patient attendances at various hospitals and clinics and some in-patient facilities are available.

A library and database is held in Glasgow and a smaller facility in London. Local medical school libraries and most local authority libraries should have a selection of books on homoeopathy. The *British Homoeopathic Journal* is published quarterly from the Faculty in London.

Appendix I. Common homoeopathic remedies used in primary care practice

Aconite (*Aconitum napellus*, wolfsbane)   Used for fear and shock, particularly when someone has had a 'nasty fright' or panic attack and may be hyperventilating.

Arnica (*Arnica montana*, mountain daisy)   A medicine for treating acute injury, it is used to heal bruises, blows, sprains and wrenched ligaments. Arnica is also suggested for people who have surgery, particularly hysterectomy and hip replacement, and also indicated during labour.

Arsenicum album (white arsenic)   The symptoms of poisoning by arsenic are diarrhoea and vomiting and marked weakness. A patient with diarrhoea and vomiting who rapidly dehydrates and becomes weak may respond to Arsen. Alb. When the similimum is correct, the diarrhoea and vomiting may be stopped with one tablet.

Belladonna (*Atropa belladonna*, deadly nightshade)   Belladonna may be useful to give at the start of a fever to abort an illness.

Chamomilla (German chamomile)   Used for restless, fretful, and vocal patients. Particularly when the child is teething and/or irritable and wants to be carried.

Ignatia (seeds of St Ignatius' bean)   The seeds contain strychnine. For acute grief, when recently bereaved in any sense, and when the emotions are very labile.

Natrum muriaticum (sodium chloride)   A remedy for oral or genital herpes. Some homoeopaths recommend using Nat. Mur. in conjunction with the nosode Herpes Simplex 200.

Pulsatilla (windflower)   Used for catarrh, repeated otitis media with glue ear, and reduced hearing. Where the nasal discharge is 'bland', i.e. does not make the nose sore, and the nose is blocked.

Appendix II. Case histories of homoeopathic treatments

Three different patients are presented, all with similar pathology, who responded to three different homoeopathic medicines. The 'constitution' is a term used in homoeopathic medicine to refer to the sum of the physical and mental symptoms plus the psychological profile. The remedy is varied according to the constitution of the patient, and so different patients may receive different remedies even if they have the same disease. However, people can be assigned fairly easily to defined groups, similar to those that doctors are already familiar with; such as introvert/extrovert or type A/B personality. The homoeopathic types are similar but more detailed.

Case 1

A lady of 82 years with a 3 year history of symptomatic obstructive airways disease. She had required admission to hospital on three occasions. She was taking inhaled ipratropium bromide, salbutamol, and high dose beclomethasone. She frequently needed oral prednisolone. She was an extremely chilly person, even wearing bed-socks in the summer. She was thin and spare and fidgeted all through the consultation. She had a nervous disposition and was a terrible worrier. Three tablets of Arsen. Alb. 10M were given. When she was reviewed 2 months later she had improved sufficiently to be using low dose beclomethasone and salbutamol only. Three years later, when she was seen for another problem, she was free from respiratory symptoms and was not on any medication.

Case 2

A 52 year old engineer who had had asthma for 4 years. His consultant had described his condition as 'drug resistant'. His meditation was; inhaled salbutamol, salmeterol, and high dose beclomethasone plus prednisolone 5 mg daily and co-amoxyclav 1 tablet twice daily. Nebulized salbutamol was often used nocturnally. His symptoms were worst at 2–3 a.m., having to sit up to breathe with any comfort. Consequently he was always tired. His peak flow never rose much above 150. He was very sensitive to noise, light, and smells. He described himself as a 'workaholic' and would easily became annoyed or lose his temper. In appearance he was extremely neat and tidy, and could not bear disorder. He also felt very chilly. As his asthma was so severe he was given a low potency homoeopathic remedy which would not overtax his system; one tablet of. Nux. Vom., 6c 3 times daily. He was reviewed in 3 weeks, and brought his daily peak flow record with him. He had stopped using his nebulizer after 3 days and had slept right through. Next he had stopped the antibiotic, then the prednisolone. His peak flow had risen to 250 and he felt he had calmed down and was easier to live with. Over the next 6 months he managed to reduce his inhaled beclomethasone dose and only had one course of prednisolone. He was advised to take the Nux. Vom. inter-mittently at the start of a cold or if he felt his asthma deteriorating.

Case 3

A 48 year old lady who ran a newsagent's shop, also with chronic obstructive airways disease. She was very overweight with a good appetite and always felt hot, sweaty, and thirsty. She was very gregarious and could always be relied upon for an opinion, but took little interest in her appearance. She was neither diabetic nor thyrotoxic. She had always been like this, it was her constitutional state. These symptoms are matched by the remedy Sulphur and she was prescribed 6c tds. She kept sporadic peak flow readings which showed a gradual rise until she was able to ride her bike again without getting short of breath.

References

Abbott, A. (1992). Europe tightens rules that govern homoeopathic products. *Nature*, **359**, 469.

Brewin, T. B. (1993). Logic and magic in mainstream and fringe medicine. *Journal of the Royal Society of Medicine*, **12**, 721–3.

Davenas, E., Beauvais, F., Amara, J., Oberbaum, M., Robinson, B., Maidonna, A., Tedischi, A., Pomeranz, B., Fortner, P., Belon, P. *et al.* (1988). Human basophil degranulation triggered by very dilute antiserum. *Nature*, **333**, 816–18.

Deklerk, E. S. M. D., Blommers, J., Kuik, D. J., Bezemer, P. D., Feenstra, L. (1994). Effect of homoeopathic medicines on daily burden of symptoms in children with recurrent upper respiratory tract infections. *British Medical Journal*, **309**, 1329–32.

Ernst, E. (1994). Researching complementary medicine. *Members' handbook 1994*, pp. 613–15. RCGP, London.

Kleijnen, J., Knipschild, P., ter Riet, G. (1991). Clinical trials of homoeopathy. *British Medical Journal*, **302**, 316–23.

Gibson, S., Gibson, R. (1987). *Homoeopathy for everyone*, pp. 102–6. Penguin, London.

GRECHO (Groupe de Recherches et d'Essais Cliniques en Homéopathie) (1989). Evaluation de deux produits homéopathiques sur la reprise du transit après chirurgie digestive. Un essai contrôlé multicentrique. *Presse Medicale*, **18**, 59–62.

Hahnemann, S. (transl. Künzli, J., Naudé, A., Pendleton, P.) (1983). *Organon of Medicine*, 6th edn, pp. 14, 26, 47. Gollancz, London.

Lokken, P., Straumsheim, P. A., Tveiten, D., Skjelbred, P., Borchgrevink, C. F. (1995). Effect of homoeopathy on pain and other events after acute trauma. Placebo-controlled trial with bilateral oral surgery. *British Medical Journal*, **310**, 1439–42.

Maddox, J., Randi, J., Stewart, W. W. (1988). 'High-dilution' experiments a delusion [news]. *Nature*, **334**, 287–91.

MORI (Market and Opinion Research International) (1989). Research on alternative medicine. *The Times*, London, 13 November 1989.

Murray, J., Shepherd, S. (1993). Alternative or additional medicine? An exploratory study in general practice. *Social Science and Medicine*, **37**, 983–8.

Reilly, D. T., Taylor, M. A., McSharry, C., Aitchison, T. (1986). Is homoeopathy a placebo response? Controlled trial of homoeopathic potency, with pollen in hayfever as a model. *Lancet*, **ii**, 881–6.

Smith, I. (1995). Commissioning complementary medicine [editorial]. *British Medical Journal*, **310**, 1151–2.

Swayne, J. M. D. (1989). Survey of the use of homoeopathic medicine in the UK health system. *Journal of the Royal College of General Practitioners*, **39**, 503–6.

Walach, H. (1993). Does a highly diluted homoeopathic drug act as placebo in healthy volunteers? Experimental study of Belladonna 30C in double-blind crossover design, a pilot study. *Journal of Psychosomatic Research*, **37**(8), 851–60.

Suggested reading

Boyd, H. (1981). *Introduction to homoeopathic medicine.* Beaconsfield, Beaconsfield.

Gibson, S., Gibson, R. (1987). *Homoeopathy for everyone.* Penguin, London.

Kayne, S. (1997). *Homoeopathic pharmacy.* Churchill Livingstone, Edinburgh.

Kent, J. T. (1986). *A repertory of the homoeopathic materia medica.* Homoeopathic Book Service, London (also available as a software package).

Murphy, R. (1995). *Lotus Meteria Medica.* Lotus Star Academy, Pagoa Springs, Colorado.

Schroyens, F. (ed) (1993). *Synthesis: homoeopathic repertory.* Homoeopathic Book Publications, London.

Vithoulkas, G. (1980). *The science of homoeopathy.* Grove Press. New York.

Useful addresses

Blackie Foundation Trust,
1 Upper Wimpole Street,
London W1M 7TD.
0171 224 1704 (telephone);
0171 224 1094 (fax).

British Homoeopathic Association,
27a Devonshire Street,
London W1N 1RJ.
0171 935 2163 (telephone).

Faculty of Homoeopathy,
Royal London Homoeopathic Hospital,
Great Ormond Street,
London WC1N 3HR.
0171 837 8833 (telephone);
0171 833 7238 (fax).

Research Council for Complementary Medicine,
60 Great Ormond Street,
London WC1N 3JF.
0171 833 8897 (telephone).

HOMOEOPATHY Homepage URL
http://www.dungeon.com/home/~cam/index.html

CHAPTER TWELVE

The future of prescribing in primary care

Richard Hobbs

As this book has demonstrated, prescribing within primary care remains a particularly complex healthcare issue. Prescribing is a high volume and high cost activity (consuming over 50% of the total expenditure on UK primary care services and some 1% of the total expenditure of the NHS).

- It requires a high knowledge base amongst clinicians, and further requires more frequent updating than any other branch of medicine.
- It is subject to close governmental intervention, in terms of the licensing and regulation of industry and the monitoring and education of clinicians.
- It is associated with sophisticated marketing of clinicians by industry, linked to highly sophisticated research and development programmes by some of the most successful commercial organizations in developed societies.
- It requires careful systems to ensure smooth operation of prescribing at the interfaces between primary care and the public, and between primary and secondary care.

Although there are numerous sources of information on the therapeutics of prescribing, many of those involved in prescribing remain less knowledgeable on the wider issues. The main aim of this book has been to address these knowledge gaps.

But what of future trends in primary care prescribing? The implications of the changes described in Chapter 2 will continue. Most governments will continue to attempt to limit the increased costs of prescribing, or (which is more relevant), maintain or reduce the proportionate expenditure on prescribing within the overall health care budgets. They will do this by extending many of the methods discussed in Chapters 8 and 9.

The actual methods of influencing practitioner prescribing are unlikely to be significantly altered from those employed today. However, the methods themselves are likely to become more sophisticated through the use of electronic feedback of information on individual prescribing practice, through the use of electronic formularies and the like. Indeed, with the advent of GP software operating systems, which provide personal computer technology at the consulting desk, there is a much greater potential for providing information on drug costs, therapeutic alternatives and management advice at the point of decision to prescribe. Electronic links between physician and pharmacist should also improve prescribing safety and simplify the prescribing process (Hobbs, 1994).

In terms of prescribing costs, any objective of containing overall expenditure on prescribing is likely to prove very difficult to realize. We know that there are many patients in primary care with chronic problems that would benefit from medication who remain undiagnosed. We are also aware that for the patients who are diagnosed, for a significant proportion their disease control remains unsatisfactory. Both of these issues are likely to increase both prescribing volume and costs, as primary health care becomes more efficient and comprehensive at case finding, and with improvements (through practice policies) in patients' adherence to therapy.

Furthermore, novel compounds are becoming ever more expensive to develop. There remains a greater imperative for a re-evaluation of licensing arrangements across countries (see Chapter 4), in an attempt to reduce the costs of developing safe and effective drugs. The greater the cost of drug development, inevitably the greater the cost of the prescription, whatever pricing arrangements that governments may negotiate with the pharmaceutical industry.

The challenge for healthcare systems is therefore how to fund an increased range of safe and effective treatments available for the total range of patients who would most benefit from therapy. Since some element of rationing for prescribing is inevitable, the more widespread of understanding and use of health economics, to assist in decisions over who should receive, what medications, and in what circumstances, is therefore appropriate. Such data will feed into practice formularies, and management guidelines and protocols.

These enhanced pressures on prescribing budgets through greater case finding should not be underestimated. Comparatively recent data upon the effectiveness of ACE inhibitors in improving the prognosis for heart failure, the reduction of strokes through the anticoagulation of patients with non-rheumatic atrial fibrillation, and the promising data on the reno-protective effects of ACE inhibitors in diabetes, are all examples of important new therapeutic indications in important and common chronic disorders.

One of the likely consequences of such changes is that the focus on prescribing will need to shift from an emphasis on costs to consideration of cost effectiveness, even though this process is likely to increase overall prescribing costs. This re-focusing on cost effectiveness will be much more achievable by clinicians and acceptable to governments if there is a greater future emphasis upon managed care programmes for chronic disorders. As was discussed in Chapter 9, managed care assumes a unified budget for all health care within defined disease groupings. Under these circumstances, it may well be more appropriate to expend a higher proportion of the overall costs in managing a condition on investigations and treatments. This pattern of care becomes appropriate when there is evidence that effective treatments reduce expensive outcomes. Clearly where these outcomes involve hospital admission or long term rehabilitation, the potential to see more cost-effective management through prescribing will be apparent.

One further aspect of some of the new drugs under development is the specialist nature of their indication. Some of these compounds would, under current circumstances, only be prescribed within in a hospital environment. However the move to more comprehensive services being available within primary care settings will continue the trend for more specialist 'drugs' being prescribed in primary care. Such developments will require better mechanisms to develop joint management guidelines across the hospital/community interface. However, it is difficult enough to develop effective guidelines and even more problematic to successfully implement them. There will need to be, therefore, much greater future emphasis upon tools that will assist the GP to prescribe specialist 'drugs' safely.

One very important mechanism is likely to be the wider availability of computerised decision support systems (DSS) which can provide automatic prompts to the point of prescribing, backed up by advisory material, in the form of hypertext. The potential for such DSS is only now becoming a reality, with data showing that computerised DSS on lipid management can improve the appropriate testing of patients with hyperlipidaemia (Hobbs *et al.*, 1996a). More recent data has further demonstrated highly significant improvements in INR control amongst patients having their warfarin monitored in primary care settings, where the dosing recommendations and recall times are calculated by a computer DSS (Fitzmaurice *et al.*, 1995). This latter example has also provided data on the wider potential for comprehensive drug monitoring in primary care through the use of near patient (or point of care) tests, alongside computerised DSS (Fitzmaurice *et al.*, 1995; Hobbs, 1996) or modification of management decisions through immediate availability of test results (Hobbs *et al.*, 1992; Hobbs *et al.*, 1996b).

Although the principal consequence of new drug development will be on the prescribing budgets in primary care, there should also be an enhanced role for primary care in the development of such novel compounds. As was pointed out in Chapter 3, more of the patient data in phase II and III drug trials could come from patients in primary care. The main advantage of research in these cohorts is the more reliable information obtainable on the sorts of patients who will ultimately be recipients of successful compounds. However, because of the requirements for close monitoring of patients, particularly in phase II, such studies require the establishment of specialist primary care drug research facilities to provide the monitoring staff, and networks of experienced practices used to working to rigid protocols. Such facilities, when they are available, can make important contributions to safer drug development (Beaumont *et al.*, 1993).

Whatever the future holds in terms of new drugs to prescribe or new regulations for prescribing practice, there will be no escaping the continued interest in prescribing across the varied groups involved in managing or delivering health care. Prescribing will continue to be the principal healthcare management activity in terms of volume, and one of the main forms of management in terms of cost. As therapeutic options become ever more sophisticated, there will need to be as great an emphasis on the technologies which support prescribing as upon the technologies that currently support drug development.

References

Beaumont, G., Gringas, M., Hobbs, F. D. R., Drury, V. W. M. *et al.* (1993). A randomized, double-blind, multi-centre, parallel-group study comparing the tolerability and efficacy of moclobemide and dothiepin hydrochloride in depressed patients in general practice. *International Clinical Psychopharmacology*, 7(3/4), 159–65.

Fitzmaurice, D. A., Hobbs, F. D. R., Murray, E. T., Gilbert Rose, P. E. (1995). A randomised controlled trial comparing primary care oral anticoagulant management utilising computerised decision support (DSS) and near patient testing (NPT) with traditional management. *Family Practice*, 12, 253–4.

Hobbs, F. D. R. (1994). *Community pharmacy links to general practice.* 15th Unichem Annual Conference, Vancouver, Canada.

Hobbs, F. D. R. (1996). Near patient testing in primary care (editorial). *British Medical Journal*, 312, 263–4.

Hobbs, F. D. R., Broughton, P. M. G., Kenkre, J. E., Thorpe, G. H. G., Batki, A. (1992). Comparison of the use of four desktop analysers in six urban general practices. *British Journal of General Practice*, 42, 317–21.

Hobbs, F. D. R., Delaney, B. C., Carson, A., Kenkre, J. E. (1996a). A prospective controlled trial of computerized decision support for lipid management in primary care. *Family Practice*, 13(2), 133–7.

Hobbs, F. D. R., Kenkre, J. E., Carter, Y. H., Thorpe, G. H., Holder, R. L. (1996b). Reliability and feasibility of a near patient test for C-reactive protein in primary care. *British Journal of General Practice*, 46, 395–400.

Appendix III. Example of PACT standard report

#00001/00001/20-02-1995/00000206l/

Prescribing by:

Dr WORKLOAD
Dr No: 123456
47 BRONCHODILATOR WAY
MYOCARDIAL INFARCTION
REFLUXSHIRE

NSA 1DS

Report to:

Dr WORKLOAD
Dr No: 123456
47 BRONCHODILATOR WAY
MYOCARDIAL INFARCTION
REFLUXSHIRE

NSA 1DS

PACT PPA

3rd quarter 1994/95

PRESCRIPTION NHS PRESCRIBING INFORMATION CENTRE
PRICING
AUTHORITY

STANDARD REPORT

BNF Version Number 26

QUARTER ENDING DECEMBER 1994

For explanatory notes and practice details, please see back page

October - December 1994

PRACTICE PRESCRIBING COSTS

		Change from last year (%)
Your practice	**£439,835**	**11**
FHSA equivalent	£490,672	7
National equivalent	£470,908	7
Your own costs	**£28,122**	**19**

Your Practice costs are **below** the FHSA equivalent by **10%**
Your Practice costs are **below** the national equivalent by **7%**

See the coloured pages for prescribing information on the treatment of depression

® PACT is a registered trade mark of the Prescription Pricing Authority

© Copyright Prescription Pricing Authority 1995

#00001/000001/20-02-1995/000002061/

THE NUMBER OF ITEMS YOUR PRACTICE PRESCRIBES

		Change from last year (%)	Prescribed generically (%)	Dispensed generically (%)
Your practice	51,746	5	58	51
FHSA equivalent	62,749	1	53	47
National equivalent	62,691	0	52	46
Your own prescribing	3,927	7	67	62

The number of items your Practice prescribed is **below** the FHSA equivalent by **18%**
The number of items your Practice prescribed is **below** the national equivalent by **17%**

PRESCRIBING BY BNF THERAPEUTIC GROUP IN YOUR PRACTICE

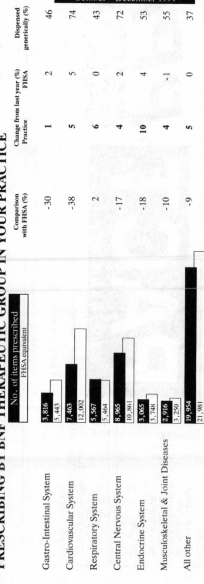

	No. of items prescribed / FHSA equivalent	Comparison with FHSA (%)	Change from last year (%) Practice	FHSA	Dispensed generically (%)
Gastro-Intestinal System	3,816 / 5,443	-30	1	2	46
Cardiovascular System	7,463 / 12,002	-38	5	5	74
Respiratory System	5,567 / 5,464	2	6	0	43
Central Nervous System	8,965 / 10,861	-17	4	2	72
Endocrine System	3,065 / 3,748	-18	10	4	53
Musculoskeletal & Joint Diseases	2,916 / 3,250	-10	4	-1	55
All other	19,954 / 21,981	-9	5	0	37

October - December 1994

3

YOUR PRACTICE'S TOP 40 BNF SECTIONS BY COST
Items and costs by section

6 October - December 1994

Ranking			Costs			Items		
			£	Compared with FHSA (%)	Last year (%)	No	Compared with FHSA (%)	Last year (%)
34	1.2	Antispasmod.&Other Drgs Alt.Gut Motility	3,332	4	16	406	22	1
1	1.3	Ulcer-Healing Drugs	50,955	-14	9	1,179	-30	8
30	1.5	Treatment Of Chronic Diarrhoeas	3,804	7	29	136	7	12
28	1.6	Laxatives	4,116	-44	12	1,076	-37	6
15	2.2	Diuretics	6,773	-18	-9	2,164	-36	1
14	2.4	Beta-Adrenoceptor Blocking Drugs	8,723	-22	-5	1,301	-28	6
4	2.5	Antihypertensive Therapy	21,635	-25	14	1,006	-37	12
8	2.6	Nitrates/Vasodilators/Ca Chann Blockers	17,632	-39	-3	1,499	-43	-6
25	2.12	Lipid-Lowering Drugs	4,221	-24	4	126	-40	21
7	3.1	Bronchodilators	18,135	-17	8	2,980	0	5
3	3.2	Corticosteroids	23,919	-17	4	1,363	-5	8
36	4.1	Hypnotics And Anxiolytics	3,115	-2	-3	1,966	-13	6
33	4.2	Drugs Used In Psychoses & Rel.Disorders	3,390	-18	-6	395	-41	0
6	4.3	Antidepressant Drugs	20,071	24	24	1,576	-9	18
35	4.6	Drugs Used In Nausea And Vertigo	3,131	-3	6	544	-13	-7
10	4.7	Analgesics	15,902	-6	-8	3,475	-21	1
20	4.8	Antiepileptics	5,734	-7	4	614	-15	-5
21	4.9	Drugs Used In Park'ism/Related Disorders	5,634	-11	25	266	-32	-1
2	5.1	Antibacterial Drugs	33,905	68	20	5,790	12	-6
32	5.2	Antifungal Drugs	3,492	33	0	209	35	-3

8 | October - December 1994

ITEMS PERSONALLY ADMINISTERED OR DISPENSED BY YOUR PRACTICE

	Personally Administered		Dispensed	
	This year	Last year	This year	Last year
Practice cost	£16,650	£9,712	n/a	n/a
- of total practice cost	3.7%	2.45%	n/a	n/a
No of items	2,510	2,161	n/a	n/a
Av. cost/item	£6.63	£4.49	n/a	n/a

Overall av. cost/item £8.50   Last years overall av. cost/item £8.03

PRACTICE PROFILE

	Total list size	Patients 65 & over	Temporary residents	No. PUs
Dr WORKLOAD	1,924	463	0	2,850
Practice	27,801	3,809	218	35,419

TOTAL PRESCRIBING ASCRIBED TO YOU

	Items	Cost (£)
Dr WORKLOAD	3,927	28,122
Trainee	-	-
Deputising services for the Practice	5	9

EXPLANATORY NOTES Please refer to the PACT/IPS Technical Guide for more detailed explanations.

FHSA Equivalent Throughout this report all figures represented as "FHSA equivalent" are based on the actual figures for the local FHSA adjusted to create an imaginary practice with the same number of PUs as your practice.

National Equivalent Throughout this report all figures represented as "National equivalent" are based on the actual figures for England adjusted to create an imaginary practice with the same number of PUs as this practice.

Change from last year The % change from the equivalent period last year.

Costs Total Net Ingredient Cost

Therapeutic Groups The six therapeutic groups listed are those which incurred the highest costs in England from April 1993 to March 1994. The term "All other" includes preparations, dressings and appliances.

New Drugs For the purposes of PACT®, drugs are classified as new for a period of three years after the receipt by the PPA of the first prescription for a black triangle drug (CSM monitored).

Leading Cost Drugs These drugs, using the names by which they were prescribed, are those which contributed the most to your costs. All presentations are added together to obtain the figure for each drug. Drugs you have prescribed using a proprietary name and for which a generic form is available, are identified by the letter G.

Prescribed Generically These figures relate to items prescribed by the approved name, even when a generic is not available.

Dispensed Generically These figures relate to items where a generic is available and the dispenser has been paid for a generic.

Total list size The total number of patients registered with the practice (including temporary residents and over 65s) as last notified by your FHSA.

Temporary Residents The list size shown for temporary residents is based on the same quarter of the previous year and is included in the total list size.

Prescribing Units (PU) Patients under 65 years of age and temporary residents count as one PU. Patients aged 65 or over count as three.

Trainee These figures represent all prescribing on your prescription forms that have been marked with a D in red ink.

Deputising Services These figures represent all prescribing by deputising doctors who have used prescription pads stamped with L and specified the senior partner number of your practice.

Personally Administered Items prescribed and administered by you or a member of your practice team and which attract payments under para 44.5 of the Statement of Fees and Allowances (Red Book).

Dispensed Items dispensed by a dispensing practice including any personally administered items.

In the near future you will receive request slips which will allow you to request full details of your prescribing in the form of a prescribing catalogue.

For more information contact: Help Desk, Prescription Pricing Authority, Block B, Scottish Life House, Archbold Terrace, Jesmond, Newcastle-upon-Tyne, NE2 1DB, Tel:(0191)2810766 Fax:(0191)2813628

© Copyright Prescription Pricing Authority 1995

INDEX